Believing IS SEEING

FOCUS THROUGH A GOD-CENTERED PARADIGM

JAMES E. CROLEY III, M.D.
EYE SURGEON

FAITHFUL LIFE
Publishers

Believing is Seeing
Focus Through a God-Centered Paradigm

Copyright © 2016 by James E. Croley III, M.D.
drcroley@floridacataract.com

ISBN: 978-1-63073-168-7

Published and printed by:
Faithful Life Publishers • North Fort Myers, FL 33903
888.720.0950 • info@FaithfulLifePublishers.com
www.FaithfulLifePublishers.com

All rights reserved. No part of this publication may be reproduced, stored in a retrieval system, or transmitted in any form or by any means—electronic, mechanical, photocopy, recording, or any other—except for brief quotations in printed review, without the prior permission of the author and/or publisher.

Published in the United States of America

19 18 17 16   1 2 3 4 5

Table of Contents

Introduction		5
1	What is a Paradigm?	7
2	My Paradigm	46
3	Looking Inside Your Brain	55
4	Seeing is Believing (Maybe?) or Your Perception	72
5	Health Benefits of a God-Centered Paradigm	90
6	Spiritual Benefits of a God-Centered Paradigm	115
7	Paradigms in the Bible	134
8	The Holy Spirit or God's Presence on Earth	158
9	Tripartite Man — Spirit, Soul, and Body	184
10	How Much God Loves You	208
11	God in Our Brain	223
12	Work, Attitude, Success, and Winning	240
13	Emotions	258
14	Meditation	269
15	A God-Centered Paradigm (Life) Place Your Life Before God	283
Epilogue		298
About the Author		303

Introduction

I decided to write this book, because I believe I can give people a new way of thinking about living the Christian life. As an ophthalmologist, I think I can add a different perspective on living a Christian life—or what I call a *God-centered paradigm*. Your eyes and brain are incredible designs and structures developed by God. The intricacy and interconnectivity of the human body is amazing.

You may have heard that you only use 10% of your brain. That is not true. Your brain is constantly processing large amounts of information and performing a tremendous number of tasks 24 hours a day. All the parts of your brain are involved with numerous connections, which you will learn about in the book. It is true that you can only store or keep in memory a very small portion of the information your brain processes each day.

One of the purposes of this book is to show you that what you are observing each and every day, may not actually be what you **think** you are seeing or observing. Because of your life's experiences, you may fail to see or perceive many things. Witnesses have been wrong about the person they identified as committing a crime. Their paradigms kept them from seeing or perceiving the incident that they witnessed.

Fortunately, the brain does not stop producing new brain cells or new pathways in the brain when you become an adult. Your brain still has *brain plasticity* or the ability to form new brain cells to learn new things. You can train yourself to see and observe things more completely or accurately. You can transform your mind, heart, soul, and spirit, which are inside you. This metamorphosis can be complete and with the proper techniques can improve your brain function, mental health, and your physical health.

I am going to give you a brief course on paradigms, brain function, and how your eyes see what they see. This book will cover what I feel is, how God changes your brain and the components that make up man and our Triune God. It will reveal to you the benefits of living a God-centered paradigm and how to change your paradigm.

God's Holy Spirit is present on earth and is everywhere. There is evidence of God's hand in every aspect of this world He created. Many people don't take the time or effort to see God in His creation. I am going to show you how your brain and vision work, so that you can learn to see this world from a new perspective. The book will give you information about the Bible's instruction, combined with my medical knowledge on living a long healthy life, centered on a Christian foundation. I quote a lot of Bible verses, because there is no better source for living your life. I combined them with medical studies and information.

I would like to dedicate this book to my mother and the memory of my father. I was very fortunate to grow up in a loving Christian family. Exposing young people to the Word of God and the grace of Jesus Christ is an important step in the path of a God-centered paradigm. I implore each one of you to be a witness for Jesus Christ to your sons, daughters, grandsons, and granddaughters at a young age. The mind is most receptive to the call of the Holy Spirit when it is young and still developing. If they are not taught and exposed to the teaching of the grace of Jesus Christ by age 12, the likelihood of them developing a relationship with Jesus is greatly reduced. There is no more important responsibility of a parent or grandparent than to be a witness for Jesus Christ to their children and grandchildren.

I would like to thank my wife Janice, who supported and helped me through the process of writing this book. It has been a wonderful learning experience. My relationship with our Triune God has been greatly advanced through studying, reading, and research. I have felt God's presence and assistance throughout the process.

Now, let's take a journey on finding your God-centered paradigm.

Chapter 1
What is a Paradigm?

One lives and analyzes data within a frame, unaware that the solution is often just outside of that frame. Never underestimate the depth of your subjectivity.
— Darrell Calkins

Christianity is not about the divine becoming human so much as it is about the human becoming divine. That is a paradigm shift of the first order.
— John Shelby Spong

Many people have heard of the word *paradigm*. You may have an idea what makes up a paradigm; but many people are not aware of how much paradigms are involved in everyday life. A good place to start is with the definition of the word *paradigm*. Here is the definition from *The Free Dictionary*.

Paradigm:

1. One that serves a pattern or model
2. A set or list of all inflectional forms of a word or one of its grammatical categories
3. A set of assumptions, concepts, values, and practices that constitutes a way of viewing reality for the community that shares them, especially in an intellectual discipline

Definition found in the *Merriam-Webster Dictionary*.

Paradigm:

1. *Example, Pattern: an outstandingly clear or typical example or archetype*
2. *An example of a conjugation or declension showing a word in all its inflectional forms*
3. *A philosophical and theoretical framework of a scientific school or discipline within which theories, laws, and generalizations and the experiments performed in support of them are formulated; broadly: a philosophical framework of any kind*

Word of origin is French and Latin from the Greek word *paradeigma* pattern and *paradeiknunai* compare.

Paradigm first appeared in the English language in the 1400s, meaning *an example or pattern*. Philosopher Thomas Kuhn (1962) has the most quoted definition of paradigm as published in *The Nature of Science Revolution*. He defines paradigm as *the underlying assumptions and intellectual structure upon research and development in a field of inquiry based at a specific point of time*. Another way of explaining a paradigm is what is generally accepted as true or fact in the world, culture, religion, science, country, or political view.

Another term that is associated with paradigm is *paradigm shift*. A paradigm shift occurs when the present set of facts, theories, observations, or perceptions are no longer correct. The single most important paradigm shift in life is when a person becomes a Christian. Many times paradigm shifts face very strong opposition from the people who are tied to the old paradigm.

Joel Barker is probably the most famous person that has written and lectured about paradigms. He used paradigms and paradigm shifts to explain how some companies succeed and others fail, based on their willingness to think outside of the box or explore new ways of doing things. People and companies fall into what is called *habituation*. Habituation is a decrease in response to a stimulus after repeated presentations. You stop paying attention to things in your environment. You take things for granted. You will read later about how your brain only retains an extremely small amount of data or information that it processes every day.

There are many examples in the business world where there were paradigm shifts. Many companies kept on doing the same old thing. They were successful and didn't need to think. They were on top of the world. But they failed to research new ways of doing things. Because of their failure to recognize new technology or a new approach in their business, they failed.

Xerox failed to shift its paradigm when it did not pursue laser printers, graphical interfaces, and Ethernet.

- In 1998, Kodak had a 170,000 employees. They sold 85 percent of all the photo paper in the world. They went bankrupt. They ignored the digital revolution. Digital cameras were invented in 1975 but had a low resolution. Kodak did not see it as a threat. It didn't take long before the resolution improved and film was done.
- Polaroid employed 21,000 people in 1978. Its instant film camera was a huge success. If you are old enough, you remember that everyone was taking their pictures with those cameras. The film would pop out of the camera and sixty seconds later you had a picture. In 1978, there were 14 million instant film cameras sold in the United States. But, Polaroid did not see the coming of the digital age and went bankrupt in 2001.
- IBM missed out when it chose in the beginning not to develop the personal computer.
- Another famous story is of the Seiko quartz watch. The Swiss are renowned for making fine intricate mechanical watches.

Their craftsmanship was beyond reproach. Swiss engineer Max Hetzel developed an electric wrist watch in 1954. But, because of the Swiss paradigm, watches had to be made with tiny intricate moving parts in order to be a real watch. They never fully engaged in the development of a simpler, more reliable, and more accurate watch. In 1974, exports of Swiss mechanical watches were nearly 45 million watches. A Japanese company called Seiko was the first company to bring to the market an analog quartz watch called the Seiko Quartz Astron in 1969. The Swiss paradigm never allowed them to grasp the shift that was occurring in the watch industry. By 1983, the numbers of Swiss watch exports fell to approximately 3 million watches.

- If Henry Ford had asked the American people what they thought about improving transportation, they would have said faster and stronger horses. Ford believed that the automobile would be the mode of transportation in the future. It looks like he was right and the general population's paradigm was wrong!

Technology is changing the way we live. Google has a computerized car that has driven across the United States without any human touching the wheel. In the future, all cars will have this technology. You just tell the car where you want to go and it takes you there. Look at some of the ramifications of that technology.

- Car wrecks will be almost non-existent.
- What will happen to car insurance? Maybe that will be gone.
- Law suits involving car accidents will disappear. No more calling an eight hundred number for a lawyer.
- No road rage!
- It will save many lives.
- That one new technology will have a ripple effect on many industries.

What is a Paradigm?

Joel Barker discusses five components to strategic exploration and anticipation.

1. Influence understanding is to understand what influences your perceptions.
2. Divergent thinking means to develop thinking skills that could discover more than one answer.
3. Convergent thinking is using thinking skills to focus integrated data and prioritize choices.
4. Mapping is important in that we draw pathways to get from present to future.
5. Imaging processes to picture words or drawings or models of the future as found in exploration.

These are important for companies, but also can be applied to our personal lives.

I got into the study of paradigms when I was on the board of the Florida Society of Ophthalmology. We were stagnating and struggling as an organization. The president at the time decided to have a board meeting, where we would try to change the direction of our organization. A company who specializes in paradigms and using their techniques with paradigms to make changes to a company or organization came to our board meeting. They have used their paradigm courses with Fortune 500 companies and had been involved with treaty agreements between countries. The course was two full eight hour days.

They spent the first four hours just describing and defining what a paradigm is. They showed many examples like the ones I briefly discussed earlier, but in more detail. They showed movies and slides. They really wanted us to get a good grasp of what paradigms are. They made it clear about how much paradigms influence everything we do in life. I am not going to take that much of your time, but I also want you to know the extent in which paradigms influence your world.

Believing is Seeing • Focus Through a God-Centered Paradigm

**I want you look at each page quickly
and go to the next page until I tell you to stop.**

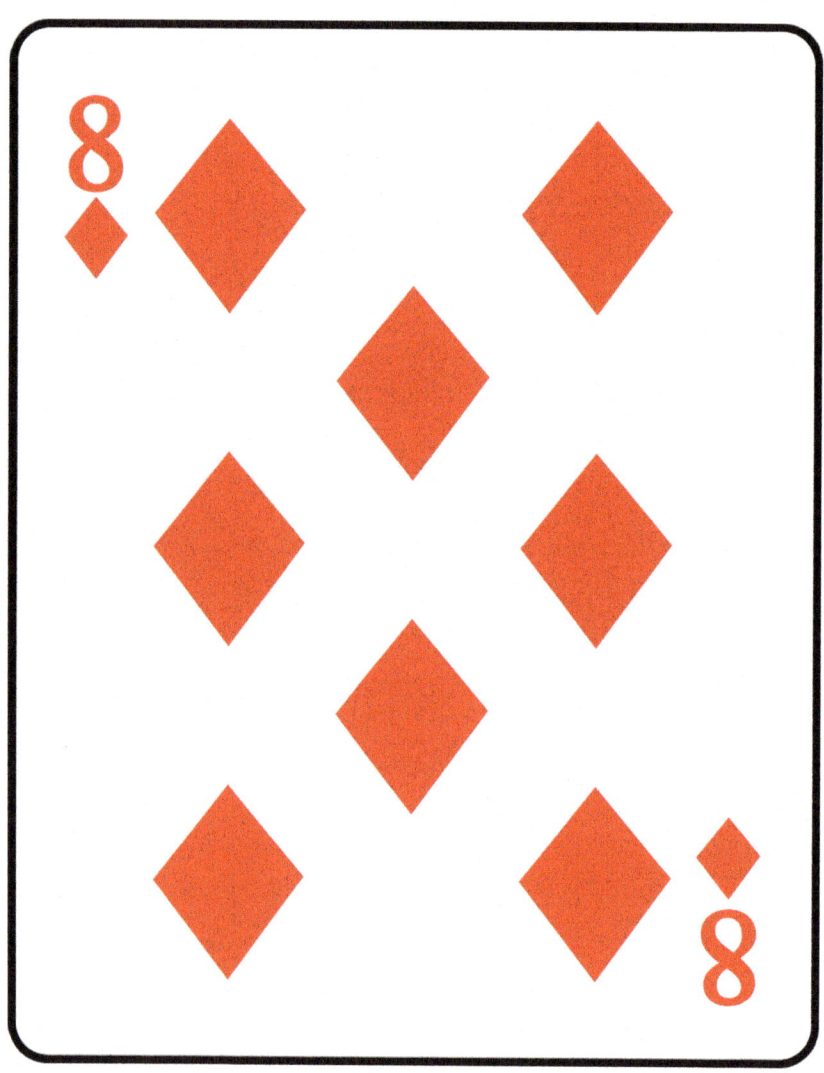

What is a Paradigm?

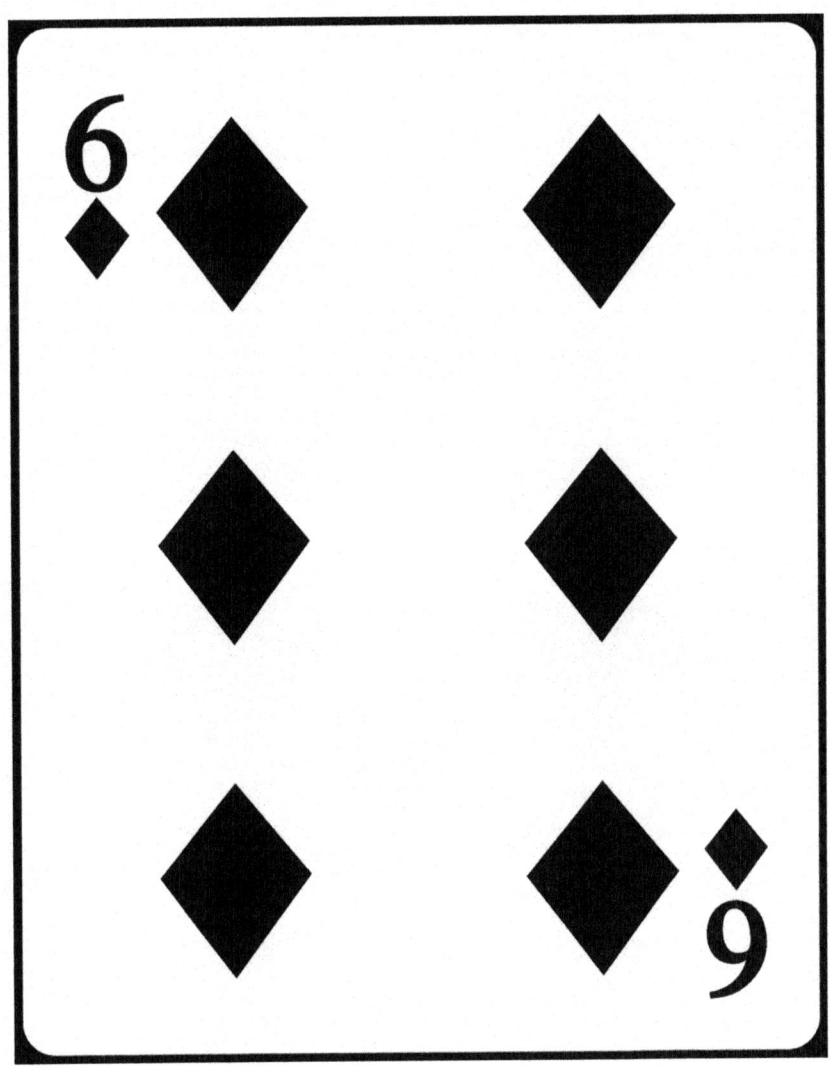

Believing is Seeing • Focus Through a God-Centered Paradigm

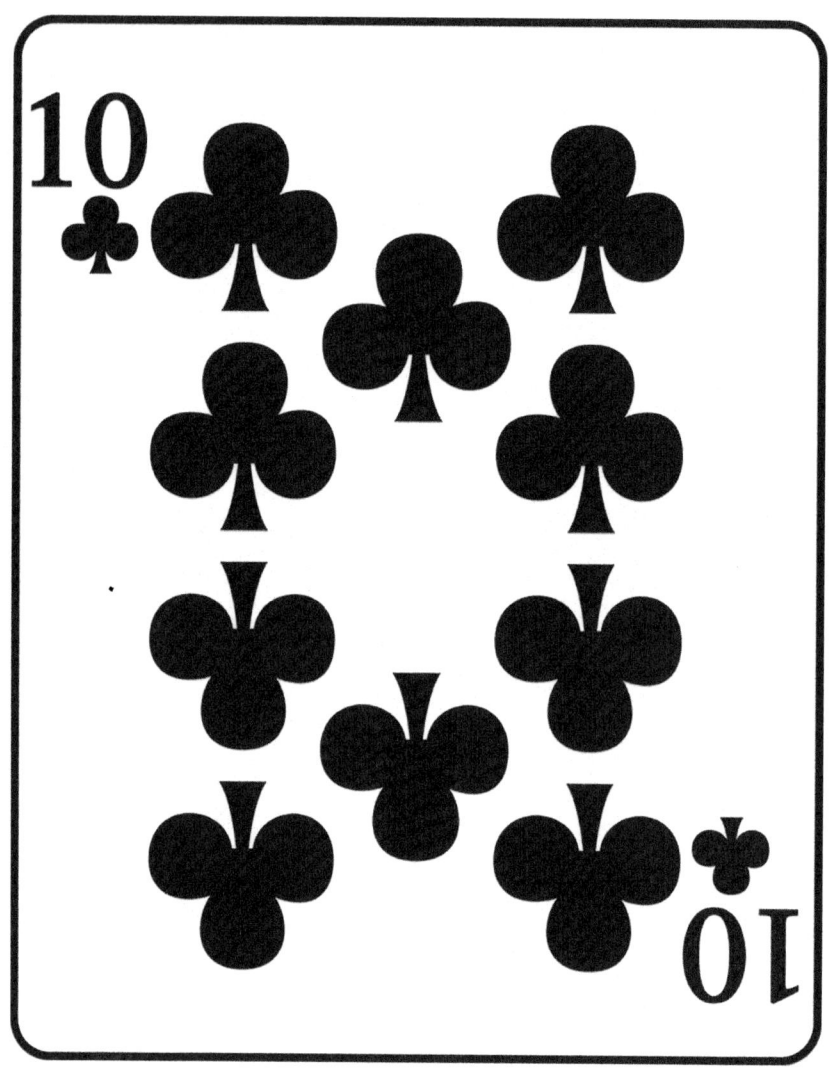

What is a Paradigm?

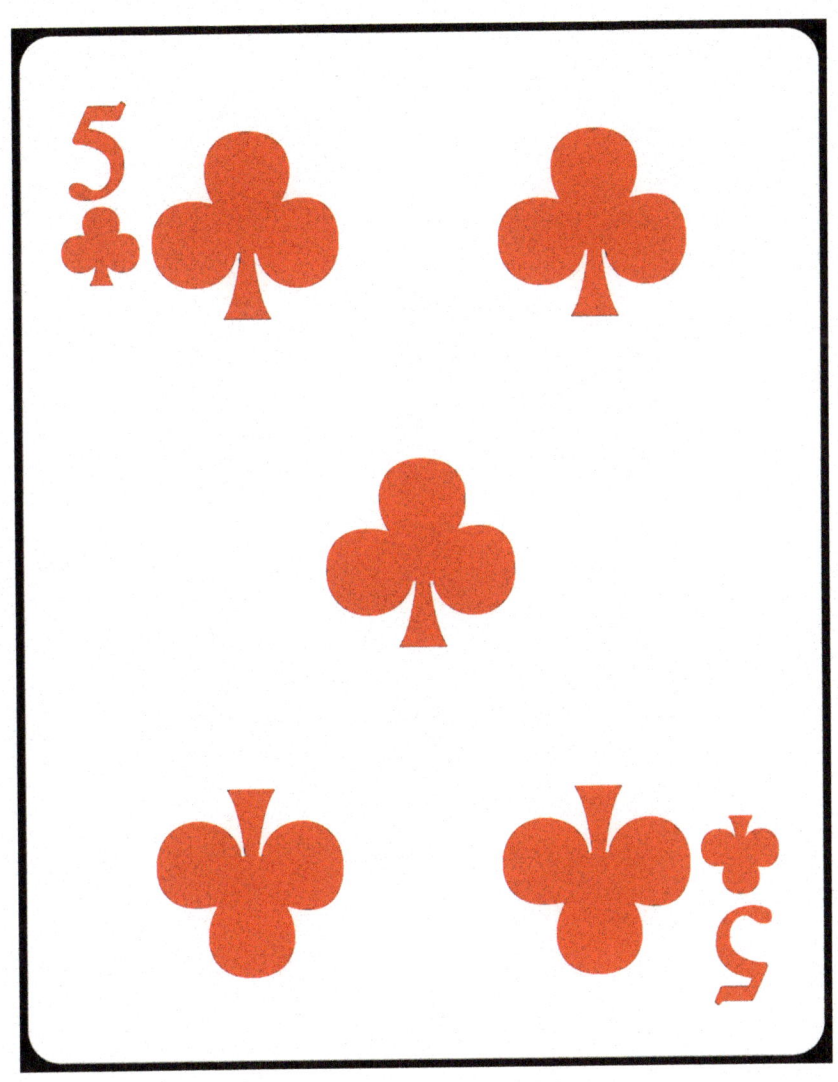

Believing is Seeing • Focus Through a God-Centered Paradigm

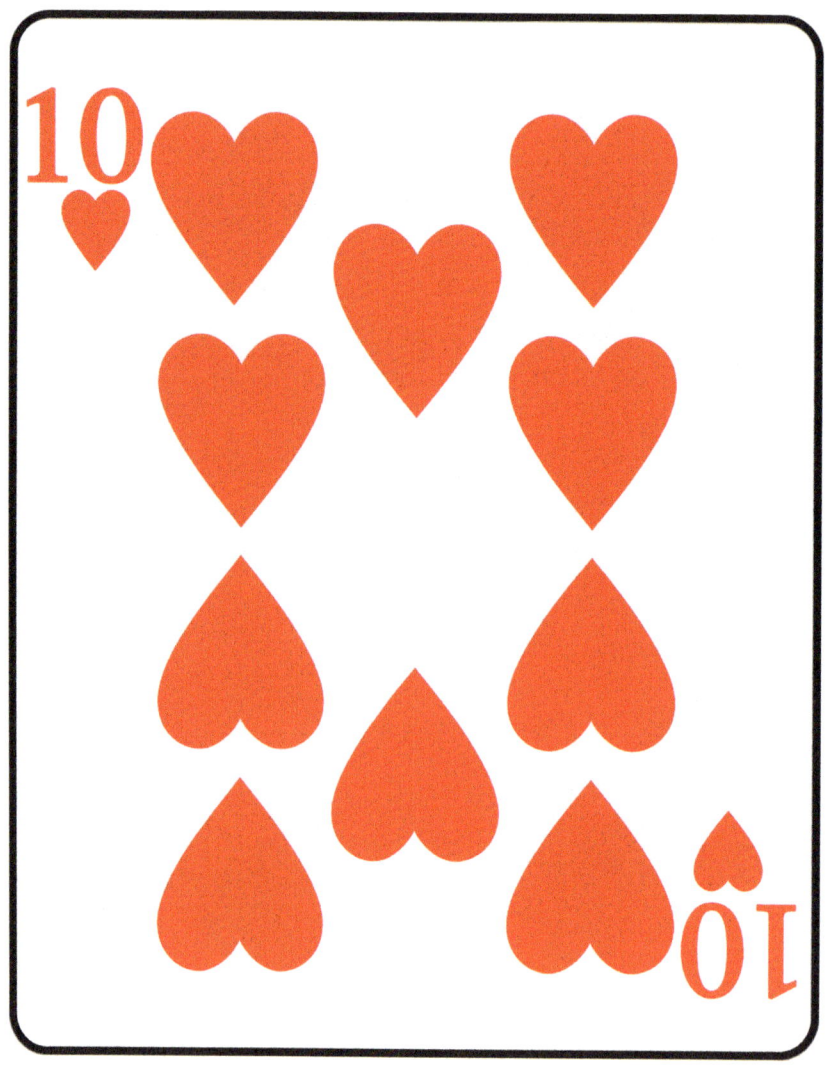

What is a Paradigm?

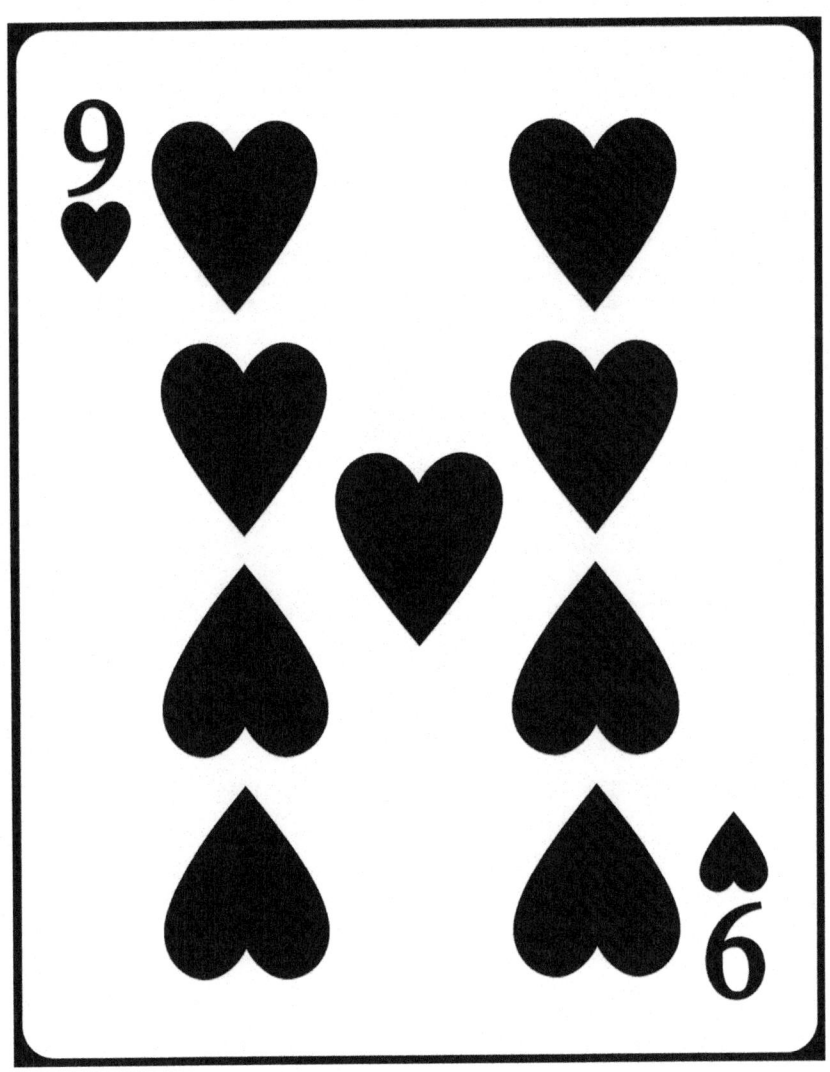

Believing is Seeing • Focus Through a God-Centered Paradigm

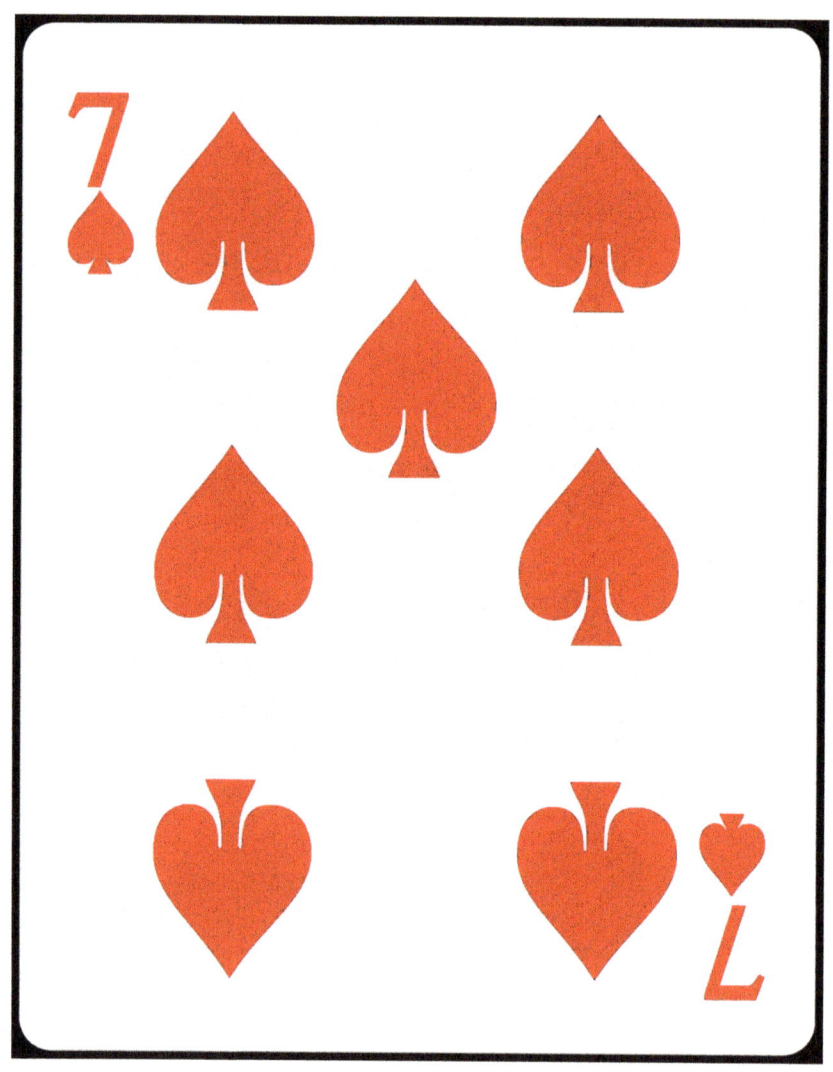

What is a Paradigm?

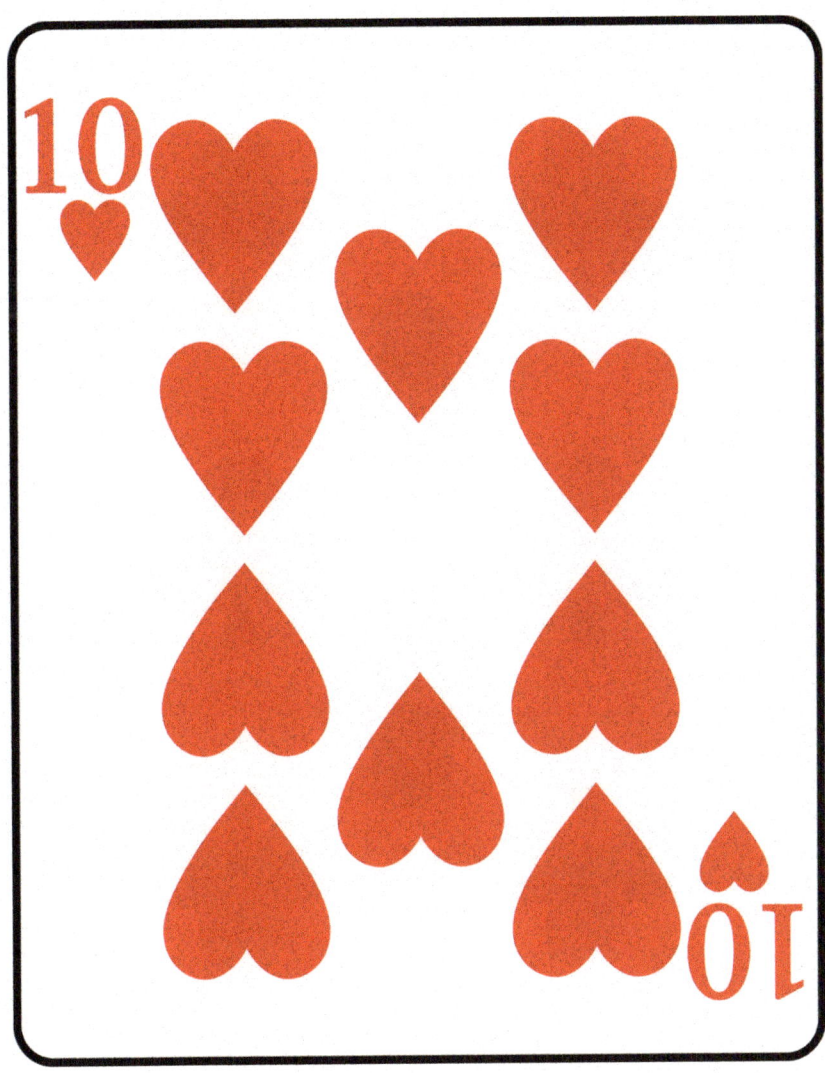

Believing is Seeing • Focus Through a God-Centered Paradigm

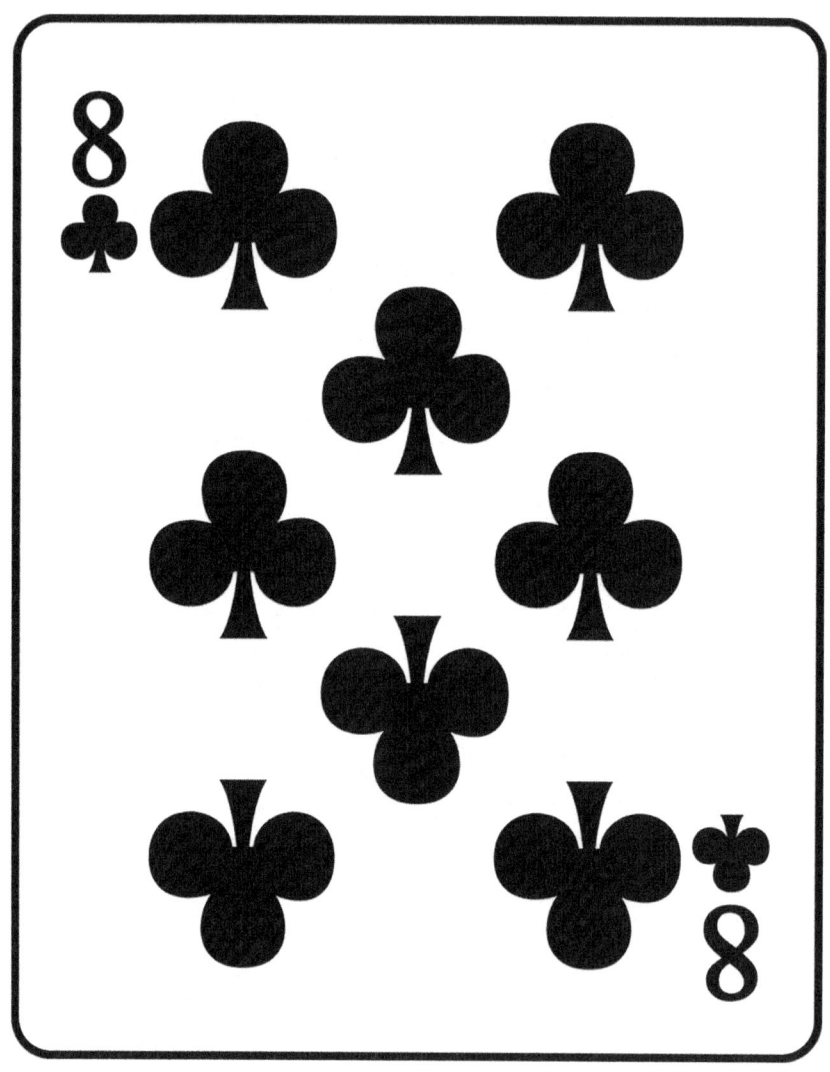

What is a Paradigm?

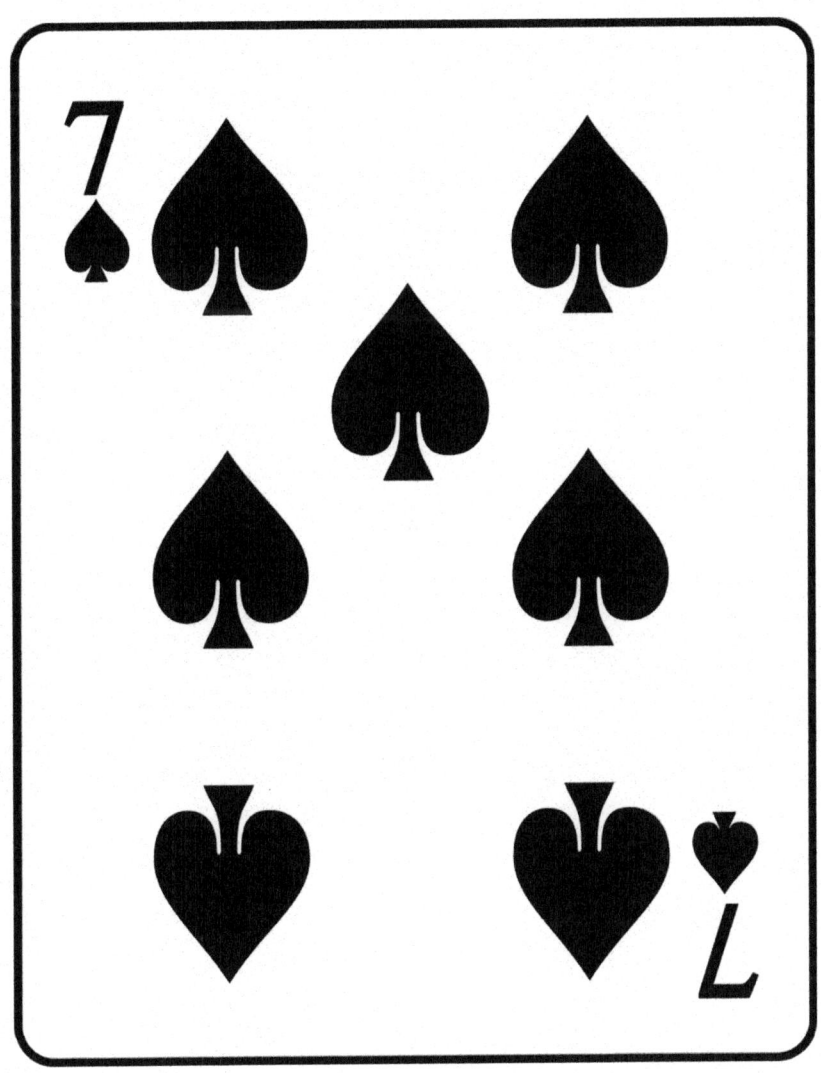

Stop
How many cards did you see?

When I give lectures on paradigms with a power point presentation, the vast majority of people count six or seven cards. With the added input of turning the pages, it may not have the same effect as watching a power point presentation. Turning the pages adds additional input to your brain processing. There were actually ten cards. Almost, no one in any lecture has counted the ten cards. The responses to the number of cards should look like a bell curve with the average number seen as ten. There should be a similar distribution of people seeing less and people seeing more than the ten cards. The reason most people don't count the correct number of cards is that four cards are the wrong color. There is no such card as a red 7 of spades or a red 5 of clubs. Even though your brain saw the ten cards, your paradigm is that there are no red spades or black hearts.

I can actually prove that the brain sees all ten cards with a test called a VEP or visual evoked potential. This test is like an EEG of the brain, except that we are only testing the brain activity in the occipital lobe of the brain. The occipital lobe is located in back portion of the brain and is the vision center of the brain. Light enters the eye and is received on the retina. The retina transmits the vision signal through the optic and out the back of the eye. The vision pathway courses all the way through the brain to the occipital lobes. The VEP measures that signal. We can tell if what a person sees reaches the vision center.

Once there, the rest of the brain gives its opinion on what is seen. The brain finally comes to a conclusion and decides what it sees based on your paradigm. I will go into further detail about how we see in a later chapter.

What is a Paradigm?

Next, let's have some fun and look at the following images. Your paradigm will determine how you see and what you perceive in the images or pictures. Look at the first image below.

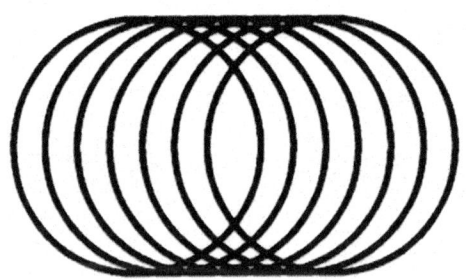

What do you see in this image? Do the rings go to the right or left? Does the direction of the rings flip back and forth from right to left? Do they predominantly go one direction or the other? Your paradigm will determine the predominant direction of the rings.

What do you see in this picture?

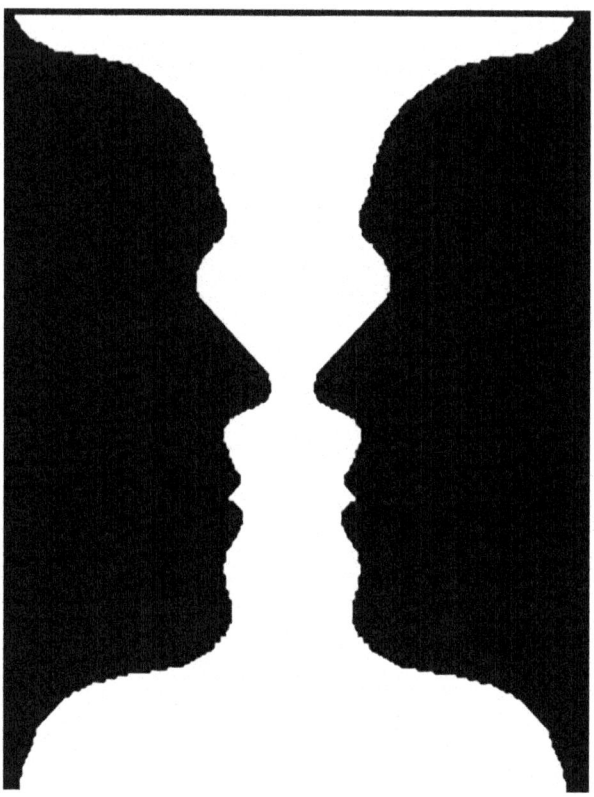

When you first look at this picture, what do you see? Do you see what looks like a candle stick holder or do you first see two people facing each other? Your paradigm determines which image you saw first and which dominants what you see.

What is a Paradigm?

Do you see the face in the beans?

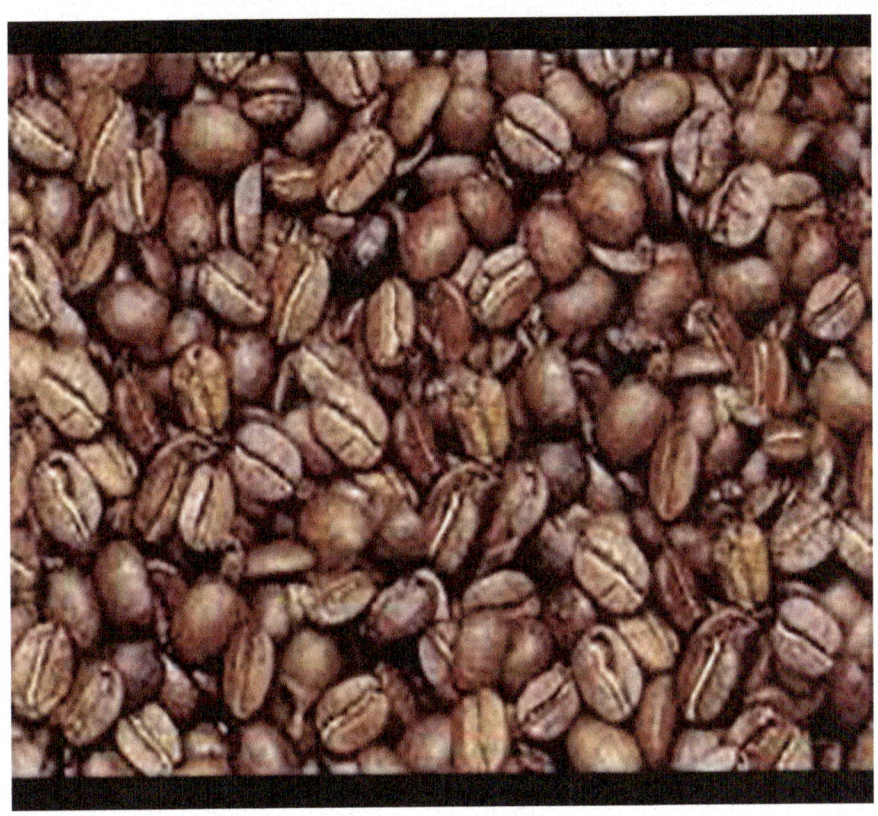

    Once you see the face, it becomes obvious. It then becomes the first thing you see when you look at the picture. For some people it may take some time and for others they find it quickly. Again, now that you have changed your paradigm with this photo, the face jumps out at you. This is how a paradigm shift works.

Who do you see in this picture? It looks like Albert Einstein. Now prop up the book and look at the picture from a further distance.

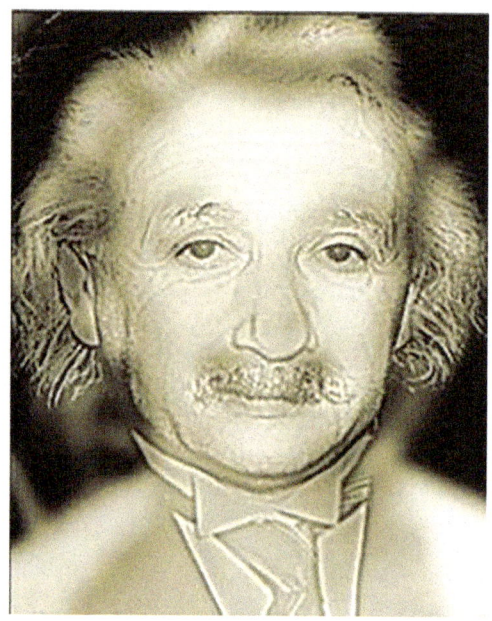

The further you get away from the picture, the more it looks like Marilyn Monroe.

Perception in life can be totally different, depending on how you observe what is happening in your life. You need to learn how to observe things from different points of view.

What is a Paradigm?

Do these lines look straight? They are straight. Take a ruler and see if they are straight.

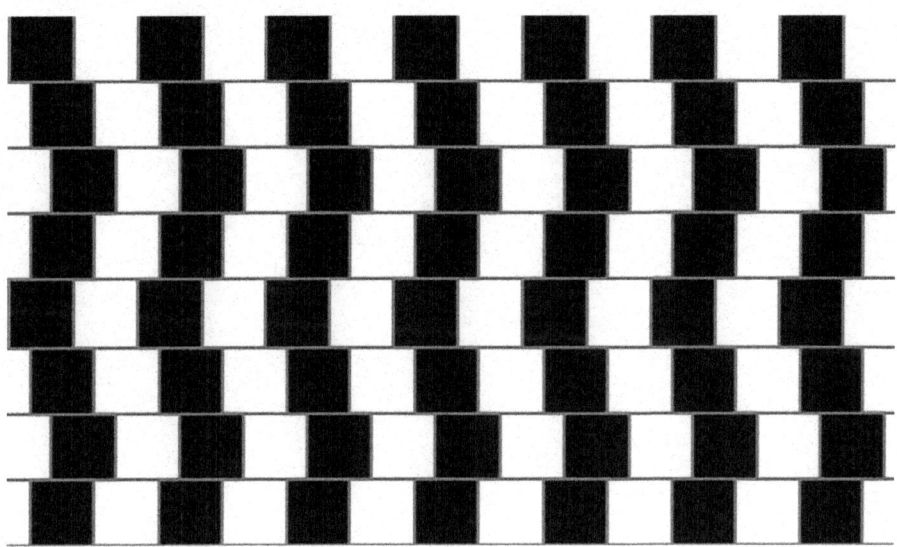

What we think we see is not always what is actually present. Your perception can be affected by many things. All your prior beliefs and experiences play a role in your perception.

What is the first thing you see here?

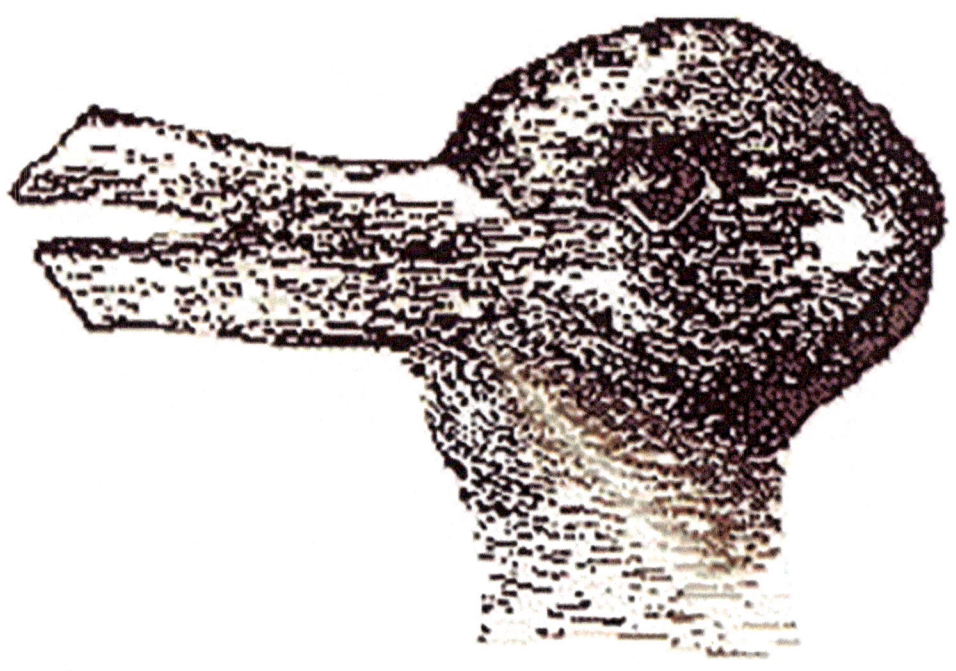

Depending on your paradigm, you may first see a duck or rabbit. You may see one of the images predominantly or it may flip back and forth.

What is a Paradigm?

What is the first thing you see this time?

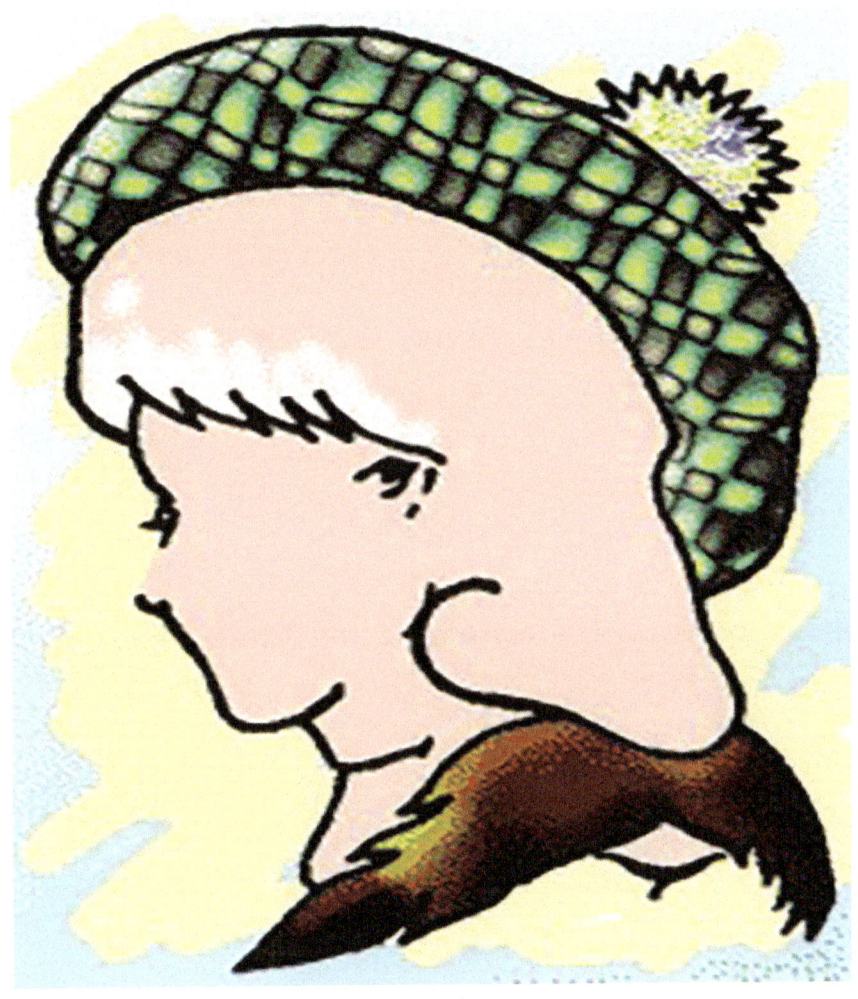

Do you see the young women facing to the left first or the older man with a large mustache facing to the right?

Are the purple lines straight or bowed in the middle?

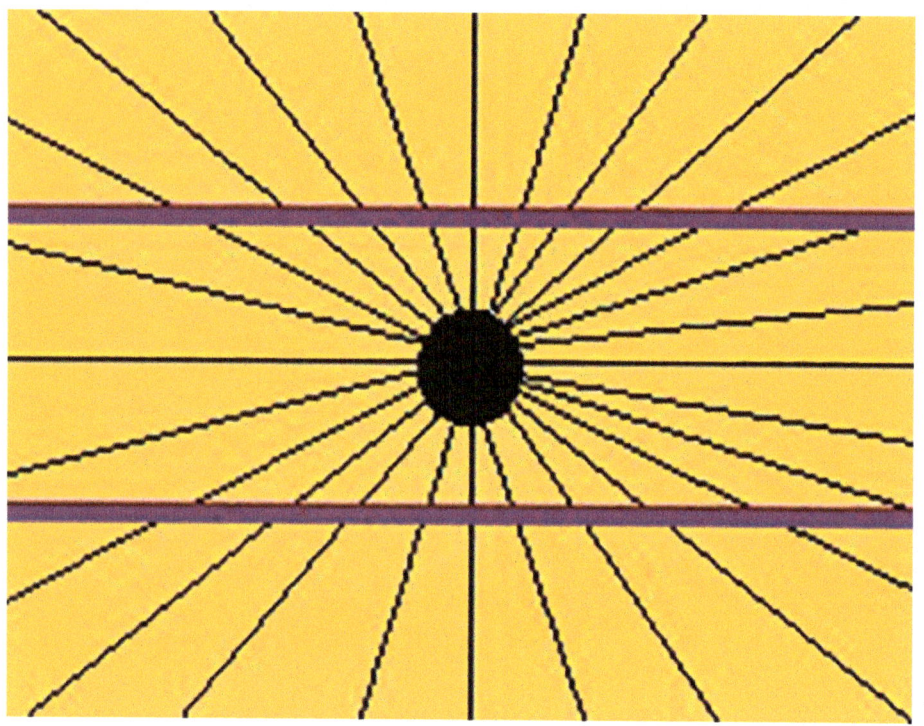

You can take a ruler and see that they are straight.

What is a Paradigm?

Let's take a look at this one. What do you see first?

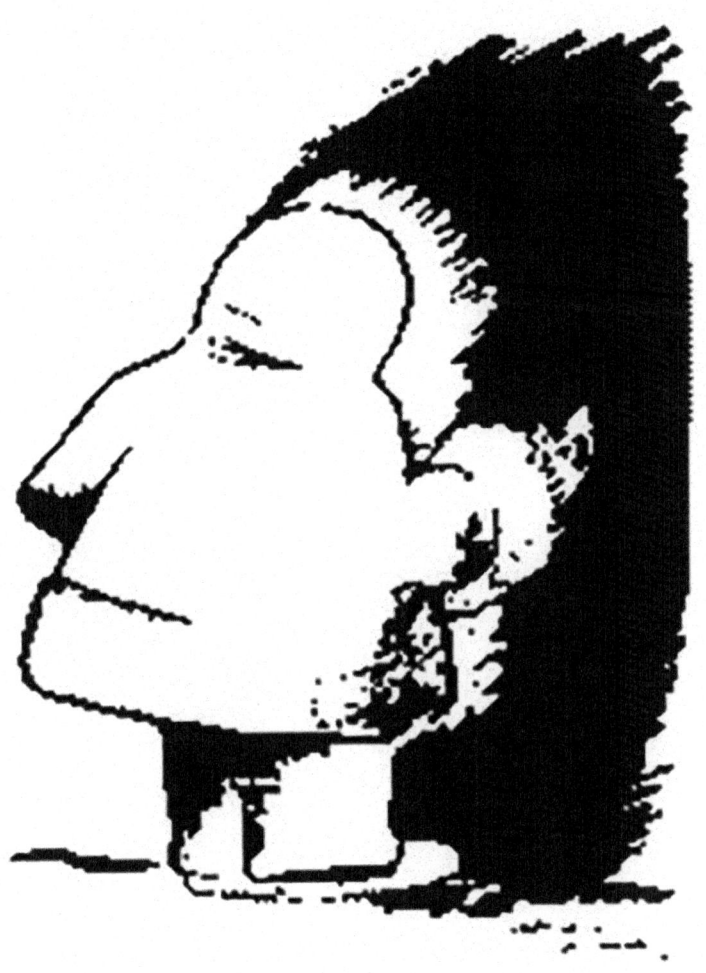

There is the face of a lady looking to the left. There is an Eskimo with their back to you looking over to the right. Are you beginning to see that depending on how you look at something, you get a very different image?

Take a look at a couple more.

What do you see this time?

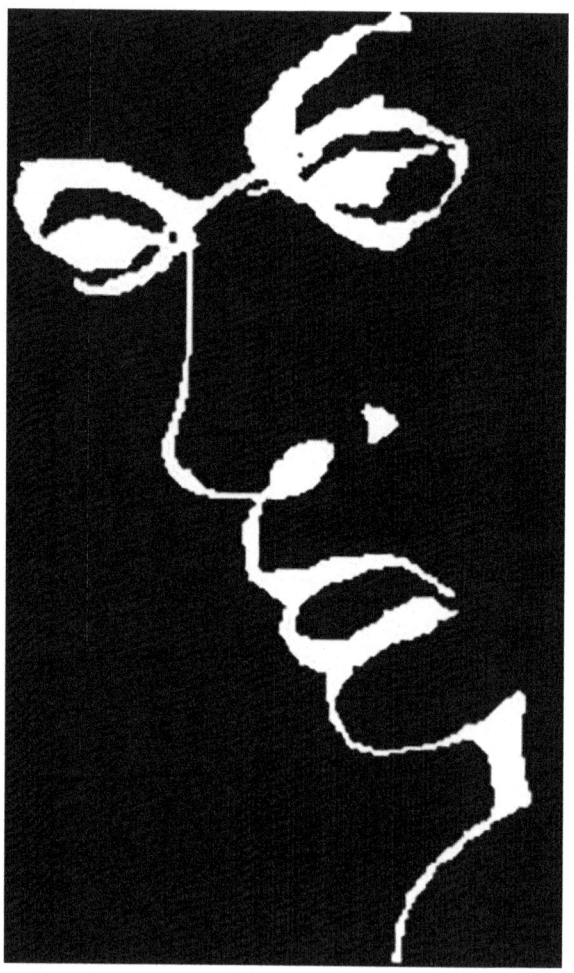

Did you only see a face or did you see the word *Liar*?

What is a Paradigm?

How easily can you say the color of the word that is written and not say the actual word. It is not that easy without some practice.

YELLOW BLUE ORANGE
BLACK RED GREEN
PURPLE YELLOW RED
ORANGE GREEN BLACK
BLUE RED PURPLE
GREEN BLUE ORANGE

Which way is the window facing when you first look at it? Is it facing right or left? Is it flipping back and forth between directions?

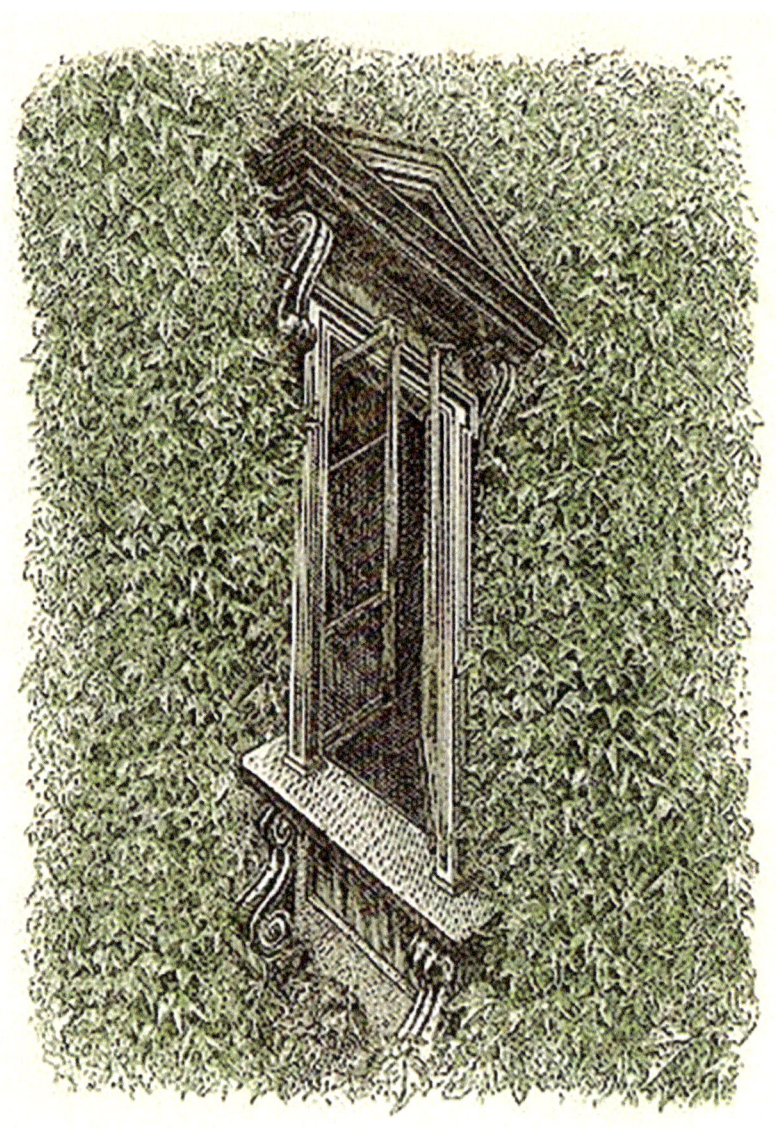

As you can see what you observe in life can be influenced by many things. Your perception and paradigm is unique to you.

What is a Paradigm?

Remember the 3D stereograms that were in the newspaper? Here is a stereogram I put together. See if you can perceive what is in the 3D image.

The best way to try and see the image is to turn the book sideways and stare above the book at a distance, then bring your gaze to the book. You almost want to try and make the image blurred, by not focusing on any specific lines or pattern in the image. Do not try to focus directly at the image.

Another technique is to start with the book close to your face. Everything is blurred when you have it right up to your face. Slowly move the book away from your face. Again, try to not focus directly at the image. The images our brain processes every second of every waking moment of the day is tremendously large. You will read later about how our brain and vision work. You can train yourself to observe your environment in a different manner than you are presently doing. Take some time and see if you see the 3D image.

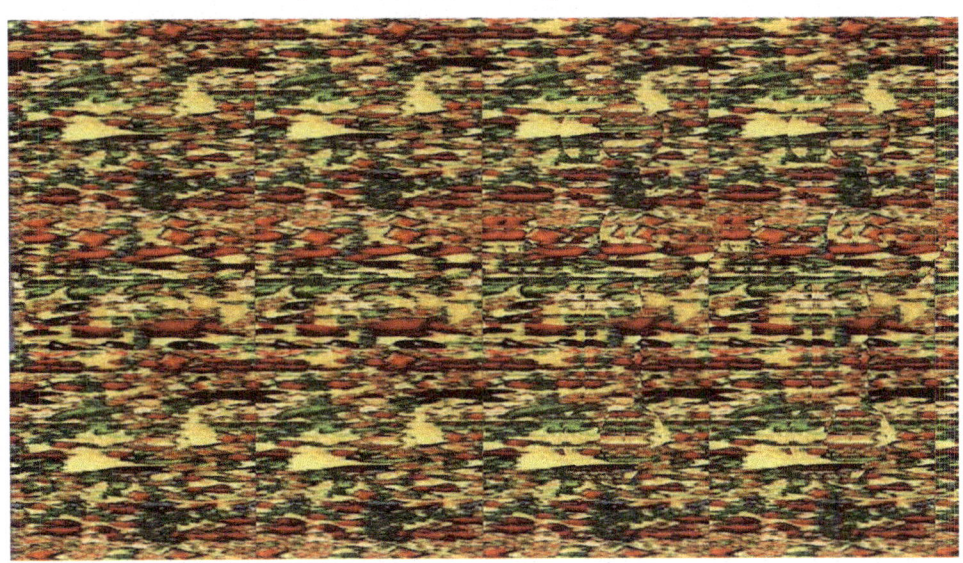

Answer: Once you see the image in 3D, you will see a cross in the middle of the picture. It has oval posts instead of a straight edged wooden cross.

Jim Wallace, who wrote the book *Cold-Case Christianity*, spoke at our church. He was a detective in Los Angeles who worked on cold cases. He relied on facts in order to solve them. In his book, he used those same detective procedures in proving who Jesus was. He talked about how he did not like eye witnesses when he was trying to solve cases. The reason—you have to vet the witness. Even if the witness is honest and telling the truth, their perception of what they saw may not be factually correct.

Unfortunately, we hear about people, who have been released from prison many years later (or worse, people have been executed), because an eye witness was wrong. If someone had been traumatized and attacked by a person, what would their paradigm be? The person who attacked them was tall, had black hair, and was somewhat overweight. What do think they will see, if they are an eye witness to another similar incident? Because of their prior experience or paradigm, they may perceive that they saw someone similar or just like the person who accosted them previously.

Many years ago eye witnesses were considered the best evidence in a case. If a witness to a crime is shown a page of pictures of the possible criminals in a case, nearly half the witnesses pick the person in the middle of the top row. Your fate could be determined by where your picture is located on the page of photos. Today, forensic evidence is much more reliable. Look at the CSI television programs that people watch today. Different paradigm!

Years ago, I had a boat and would go tarpon fishing around the waters of Southwest Florida. Depending on the time of year, I would fish off the coast of Sanibel and Ft. Myers Beach. Tarpon usually travel and stay in schools. So, once you find them you have a good chance of catching one. As they swim around, they occasionally come to the surface and roll up out of the water, sort of like a dolphin. They have very white sides that shine, especially in the sun. You can see that from a long distance away, if the water is not too rough. An experienced tarpon hunter may see the fish as much as one or more miles away.

I have taken many friends tarpon fishing to catch the famous king of fish. They are excited to get the chance of catching one of these magnificent fish. It is very exciting having a one hundred plus pound fish on the end of the line. Once hooked, they jump high out of the water, do flips and turns in the air.

As we motor around the Gulf of Mexico stalking these fish, I ask my fishing partners to look for the flash that you see when one of the tarpon rolls on the surface. Many times they never saw a fish for the whole trip, even though I had spotted many of them. I would point out the direction and distance to my fishing partner and it still did not matter. Until we actually catch a fish, they are sure that I am just telling them a story about seeing fish.

Occasionally, someone would spot a fish close to the boat. It is amazing that, from that time forward, they were able to help me see new tarpon. They have a new paradigm related to recognizing what the tarpon flash looks like. Their vision didn't suddenly improve. Their vision is just as good as mine, but I have a different paradigm. I can see a tarpon rolling on the surface a mile away. Many of my friends that I have taken tarpon fishing never see the tarpon rolling on the surface. For some, they are able to see the tarpon before the day is over. They have a paradigm shift and they can see a tarpon mile away.

Another example of a paradigm is about my wife Janice. Janice and I went bonefish fishing in the Bahamas. She told me that she enjoyed fishing and is a pretty good fisherwoman. But she had never been fishing for bonefish. Bonefish fishing is similar in a way to tarpon fishing, in that you are stalking the fish. Once you spot them, you cast your bait or lure a short distance in front of them. This is called sight fishing. The difference between bonefish fishing and tarpon fishing is that you are in very shallow clear water, sometimes only one foot deep. The guide and I would tell Janice that there were four bonefish just twenty feet away, right in front of the boat. Unfortunately, she could never see them. We caught several bonefish that day and she never saw one fish.

Now, Janice has great vision—she can spot a piece of lint on my sport coat a mile away! It is amazing that she can see something that small and at a considerable distance. But, she couldn't see a six-pound bonefish in only several inches of clear water ten feet away. Now, that is a paradigm. She has a great fine-tuned paradigm for lint!

Now, I am going to tell a story about my vision. When I do the cooking and am cleaning up after dinner, I clean the counter top. But, I never clean the counter top correctly. The moment that I am finished, she tells me I missed a spot. Now, she is across the room. I ask her where? Of course, she tells me that is right in front of my face. I look and see nothing but a clean counter. I start looking at different angles and finally when the light is just right, I see the tiny spot. I have no paradigm for seeing missed spots on the counter!

A huge paradigm for centuries was that people believed the Earth was flat. Actually, there were a variety of people centuries ago who figured out that the world was round. Most of the people did not believe that the world could be round—it was flat. If you sailed too far, you would fall off the Earth. You would be devoured by sea monsters.

Eratosthenes, a Greek astronomer, in 300 B.C. mathematically proved that the Earth was round. He calculated the curvature and size of the earth within 2 percent of the correct amount. But he was not believed by many people. Christopher Columbus furthered the theory that the Earth was round by his voyages. Ferdinand Magellan is credited with sailing around the world and proving that it is round in his voyage from 1519 to 1522. Here is some trivia for those who are into trivia. Even though he is credited, he did not finish the voyage as he was killed in the Philippine Islands in 1521. Juan Sabastian Elcano and the remainder of Magellan's crew finished the circumnavigation of the Earth. The first photographic evidence of the Earth being round was in 1946.

Another interesting story and an example of how paradigms work is the story about the blind men examining an elephant. The story of the blind men and the elephant originated in India. There are a variety of versions of the story. The story goes that there were six men who were born blind in this village. These men were watched over by the people of the village to protect them from any harm or danger.

The men heard stories about elephants and became curious. What were elephants really like? They were told how large they were, how powerful they were, and how loud they were with their trumpet calls. The men would argue back and forth about elephants. One would say that they are powerful giants. The next man would say that they are kind and gentle giants, since a princess could ride on its back. The next man would argue that an elephant is very dangerous, as it can pierce through a man with its sharp horn. The next man says that all of them are wrong—they are just a big cow. And finally one of the men said that elephants don't even exist.

Finally, the villagers got tired of their arguing and made arrangements for the blind men to meet an elephant. The first blind man touched the side of the elephant and stated that it was huge and smooth like a wall and said it must be very powerful. The second blind man touched the elephant's trunk and said it was like a giant snake. The third blind man touched the hard pointed tusk and said that the elephant is sharp and deadly as a spear. The fourth blind man touched one of the elephant's legs and said it was a large cow. The fifth blind man touched the elephant's ear and said the elephant is like a huge fan or magic carpet that could fly. The sixth blind man touched the elephant's tail and said that it is just like a piece of rope. So now the blind men are still arguing over what is an elephant.

This a great example of how a paradigm works. Each person has their own set of experiences which totally determine how they evaluate everything in their lives. You can see that our paradigms can lead to the wrong conclusion.

I have a friend who is in the FBI. I was talking with him about this book concerning paradigms and perceptions. He immediately responded that he totally understood the concept. In the FBI they are trained in how to increase their perception. During one class, a person suddenly charged in. He fired a gun with a blank at one of the students and ran out.

The instructor calmed everyone down and told them this was a test. He wanted them to write down everything they noticed about the incident. They were to provide a description of the man. Were there any distinguishing marks—even to the color of his eyes? What he was wearing? Was he right or left handed? What kind of gun did he use? Everything they could think of was to be included in their report.

When they were being trained on surveillance, they would have to train themselves to be observant about everything. If they were shown a scene on a street, they would be asked everything about that scene. For example, how many cars were on the street? What was the license number of each car? How many people were on the street? What was their descriptions, and so on? Just like the people in the FBI, you can train yourself to begin to look at your world differently.

Kenneth Boulding stated that no matter how much you study the future, it will always surprise you. But you needn't be dumbfounded. Here are some of his observations about paradigms:

- Our perceptions of the world are strongly influenced by them.

What is a Paradigm?

- Because we become so good at using our present paradigm, we resist changing them.
- It is the outsider who usually creates new paradigms.

Practitioners of the old paradigms, who choose to change early to the new paradigm, must do so as an act of faith rather than as a result of factual proof; because there will never be enough proof to be convincing in the early stages. This is just like what is in the Bible about having faith. The first step in becoming a Christian is having faith that Jesus Christ is your Lord and Savior. Then you are able to shift your paradigm around your faith in God. You then mature as a Christian, as you have a new perspective or paradigm.

Those who change to a successful new paradigm gain a new way of seeing the world. They have new approaches for solving problems as a result of the shift to the new rules. A new paradigm puts everyone back to zero. Practitioners of the old paradigm, who may have had great advantage, lose much of their leverage.

In turbulent times practice paradigm pliancy.

You have heard the saying, *You don't know what you don't know.* Another perception is, *You don't see what you don't see.* I have heard many interesting stories from my patients who have had cataract surgery. They have gradually lost their vision and are not aware of how much in many cases.

I had a nice lady who lived out in the middle part of the state of Florida. She did not have easy access to doctors. She let her cataracts advance to the extent that her vision was very poor. The day after her surgery, she was shocked when she looked into the mirror. She nearly didn't recognize that person. She told me she called her sister who lived nearby and told her off. She told her that she should be ashamed that she let her walk around looking how she looked!

I have people who told me that they bought new furniture and were upset after their cataract surgery. They thought they had purchased a particular color, but now realized it was a totally different color.

Another gentleman told me that he collected antique napkins and had purchased a set of napkins on eBay. When they arrived he was upset because they were yellow and discolored. He wrote a nasty email to the person who sold him the napkins. The following day I did his first cataract. The day after his surgery, he was getting ready to pack them up to return them. He noticed that they were perfectly white. He had to write an email to the seller apologizing for his mistake.

Your present paradigm determines what you perceive, understand, react to, and occurs in your life. As with the FBI, you and I can train ourselves to observe and perceive things differently. I am able to look at the macula in the retina and see subtle differences in the beginning stages of macular degeneration. You would not be able to see it. A radiologist trains themselves to see subtle differences on X-rays, MRIs, and CTs. You would not be able to see it, until the doctor pointed it out. Everyone's vision is the same, but their paradigms are different.

I started out with a simple definition of what a paradigm is. I hope that you are now beginning to understand how paradigms affect everything in your life.

Everything that you study, read, observe, listen to, events in the world, see on TV or instances that happen to you shape your paradigm. Your approach to each of these also shape your paradigm. You have control over what you choose to read, listen to, watch, or study. You have control over most things that influence your paradigm. In tragic events such loss of a loved one, illness, traffic accidents, and these types of instances you don't have control over them happening. But, your paradigm will determine how you respond to them.

Everyone's paradigm is unique to them. Even identical twins will not have exactly the same paradigm, because their experiences will differ.

What is a Paradigm?

They may have many similarities, but still will be their own unique person. It really is true that what information you put into a computer system and/or person will determine what comes out. Study after study is now showing that what you watch and observe in life changes people. This is especially true for children. It is very important that parents monitor what their kids are into and watch on TV.

A country has a paradigm as well. This country was founded on Judeo-Christian values. Our Constitution, laws, moral standards, and ethics were based on those values. The government, Hollywood, and the major news outlets are on a mission to change this country's paradigm. If you look back just a few years, the movies from Hollywood, the programs on TV, and the new laws that are being passed by our governments would have not seen the light of day. Now, it is accepted as normal.

The country's paradigm is changing and not for the better. Even our president has said that we are no longer a Christian nation. We as individuals need to center our lives or paradigms on God. Then we can push for a revival in America. We can then change America back to its original values. It starts with individuals. It is one person at a time until the majority of Americans take our country back.

How do you change paradigms in your life, business, or organization? I will go over it in more detail in a later chapter. You can change how you perceive and understand events and things in your life. Just like the FBI students, you can learn to look at things differently.

When you see an event, talk with someone, read a book, or other activities in your day, think about it from a different approach. What is not obvious or hidden? Why is this fact or statement being presented? Who is presenting it? Do they have a hidden agenda? There are the five Ws in evaluating a circumstance or event. I am going to add a couple more questions to think about, as well.

- Who did that?
- What happened?
- When did it take place?
- Where did it happen?
- Why that happen?
- Is there a hidden agenda?
- In what environment or circumstances did it happen?
- Observe everything.
- Listen.
- Don't narrow your focus too soon.
- Bring out the Sherlock Holmes in you.
- Is there something that does not make sense?
- Remember the TV show Lost in Space, where the robot would say, "Does not compute?"
- Don't take things on face value.

Major news networks always present their information with a significant bias or have an underlying reason for what they are reporting. Many times they take things out of context to suit their agenda. They are good at hiding their opinions.

When I was an intern, I spent two months on a cardiology rotation. The cardiologist that I spent the most time with advised me to read Sherlock Holmes books, because they would help me learn how to be a better clinician. Many times you have to be an investigator in order to find the etiology of a disease.

Sir Arthur Conan Doyle was a British writer and ophthalmologist. No wonder I like him. He wrote fifty-six Sherlock Holmes stories. As I am sure you know, Sherlock Holmes is a fictional British private detective. Sherlock Holmes' primary detection method is abductive and deductive reasoning. The Holmesian method consists primarily of observation-based inferences and observation of small seemingly insignificant clues. Holmes was always observing the dress, attitude, style and state of wear of clothes, skin marks, stains, state of mind, and physical condition in order to gain clues. The Sherlock Holmes books are a necessary read for all physicians.

Your paradigm is really who you are. How you see things, perceive, deduce, and react to things is unique to you.

We all miss many things in our lives because of habituation. We get used to a routine. The most important thing is to tune your paradigm to God's wave length.

Have some fun and start looking at things differently. You might be surprised on what you may find or what you missed that was right in front of you.

A new paradigm is waiting for you!

Chapter 2
My Paradigm

Deuteronomy 4:9 NLT

*But watch out! Be careful never to forget
what you yourself have seen.
Do not let these memories escape
from your mind as long as you live!*

I was born in the Appalachian Mountains of Eastern Kentucky in the town of Pineville. It is a giant metropolis with a population of 2,803. I was very fortunate to grow up in a Christian family who attended the First Baptist Church of Pineville. At age 7, after a church service, I told my parents I wanted to become a Christian. My mother made an appointment for me to meet with the pastor the following week. He went over what was required to become a Christian. He read several verses from the Bible and we discussed what they meant. For about thirty minutes, he asked me questions about my beliefs and faith in Jesus. I professed my faith in Jesus to him and he ended the session with a prayer. At the end of the next church service, I went forward and pronounced my profession of faith in Jesus.

I was baptized on March 8, 1958. Once I came up out of the water, I felt different. Ever since that time I have had this sensation or presence of what I assume was the Holy Spirit. I felt like I had the protection of God or I had this sensation of being safe, in a feeble way that an eight-year-old could understand. When I was young, I didn't pay too much attention to it, but I always had that feeling in the back of my mind. I was too busy growing up and having fun to pay too much attention to it on an everyday basis.

When I was twelve years old, I decided to ask the best-looking girl in school out on a date. I was going out on a limb, as it might get a little embarrassing. She was in the grade ahead of me. I was going after the best looking girl and she was older! What was I thinking? This was a big risk for a young boy, asking someone like her for my first date. I could end up being horribly embarrassed. At that age, I thought this could possibly be a disaster.

She accepted and I was thrilled. We were going to a party for kids at the church. Therefore, my parents were OK with me going on a date at this age. My dad drove us to the church and picked us up after it was over. That was my first and last date with her. The following year she was in high school and had all the older boys dating her. I had no chance, as I was too young to drive a car. It turns out that I was too busy anyway—sports, class work, and other activities.

I made the decision that I wanted to be an ophthalmologist at age fourteen. I knew that I had a long tough road ahead of me and dating was secondary. I went to all the dances at school, but never got seriously involved with anyone. I had my dream that I wanted to accomplish and I was determined to see it through.

There was a small teen center in the basement of the Methodist church where kids could go after a home football or basketball game on Friday nights. There were not many things to do in our little town in Eastern Kentucky for fun. This was a safe place for kids to hang out. I was now a junior and played on the basketball team, which in Kentucky is the sport of the state. Go Big Blue! One Friday night in January, I was at the teen center after the basketball game talking with friends. What happened next is any teenage boy's (or for that matter, probably any male's) dream come true. (I know it may be common place today. but not in the sixties). The gorgeous girl of my dreams that I went out with when I was twelve came up to me. She asked if I would like to go the neighboring town with her and a couple of friends. They were going to go to a bootlegger to get some beer.

Even though Kentucky is the home of bourbon, many of the counties in Kentucky do not allow the sale of alcohol. If someone wanted any alcohol, they had to drive to a *wet* county to buy it or go to the local bootlegger. Of course, there was always the choice of buying moonshine, as well.

After she asked me, I sat there in shock. She came to me and asked me to go with her! I *had* scored a lot points in the game that night. I guess I was back on the desired list. I remember staring at her, thinking how fantastic it was that she was asking me. Out of nowhere a tiny voice in my head (or maybe it was a thought that popped into my mind) said, "Don't go." What? Really, don't go? She is beautiful and she is asking me. I sat there in a daze looking at her, saying to myself, *but I want to go*. Again, I heard a voice or that thought that I don't want to sense again say, "Don't go."

It seemed like an eternity as I sat there gazing into her eyes. Those beautiful eyes were winking at me, and her beautiful smile that would melt any heart was smiling at me. But again, those nasty words, "Don't go." It seemed like time was standing still and an eternity was passing by as I sat there trying to decide what to do. I finally looked up at her said that I was not going to go. I was totally deflated. She turned and walked out the door with three other friends.

I sat around for an hour or so and finally decided to go home. When I walked through the kitchen door, my parents were sitting there with a worried look on their faces. They had never stayed in the kitchen waiting on me to come home. They both jumped up and ran over to

My Paradigm

hug me. Wow, what did I do to deserve this attention? This must be my special night. Then, they told me that a terrible accident had occurred.

About ten minutes after she left the teen center, the girl I had so much wanted to date lost control of her Corvair. She ran head on into an eighteen-wheeler. Four of my friends were instantly killed, with one of the boys being decapitated.

The Jaws of Life had not been invented yet. It took them a long time to get them out of the car. There were no cell phones either. The ambulance driver called the hospital emergency room to give a report on the accident on his CB radio. The emergency room was covered by the local doctors in town. The doctors would take turns taking calls for the emergency room, as there were no emergency room doctors at that time. They would drive to the emergency room when needed. From there, rumors rapidly spread around town with parents calling other parents.

It was not known who was actually in the car with her. The bodies were severely injured from extent of the damage to the Corvair from the large transfer truck. The rumor was that I was in the car. I had a very similar yellow Gant shirt as one of the boys in the car that they could not identify. That was the reason for my parent's reaction when I entered the kitchen. They were so relieved that I was not one of the kids in the car.

We sat down and discussed what had happened. My parents wanted to make sure that I was going to be OK. I was in shock and did not tell my parents that I had nearly been in the car. The town and the kids at school were devastated. I was a pallbearer at three funerals on three straight days that week, including her funeral. It took a long time for things to return to a semblance of normal in our small community.

I thought that I was just lucky. I had dodged a bullet. It just wasn't my time. As a teenage boy, you think you are invincible or Superman. You sometimes do not grasp the reality of the situation. I put it in the back of my mind that a thought or voice had told me not to go. I knew that God had intervened in my life; but the memory of the incident was painful and I didn't dwell on it too much. He had protected me for the plans He had for me in the future. I tried to move forward with my life, think about my goals, my future, and keep a positive attitude. Life eventually returned to normal.

Following my freshman year of college, a group of my friends from Pineville and a couple of new friends from college decided to rent a house on the beach in Pawley's Island, South Carolina. There were eight of us piled into two cars. I was riding on the passenger side of an El Comino, with a friend of mine in the middle. A new acquaintance from college was driving his truck. I never fall asleep in a car or plane, as I enjoy seeing the countryside pass by.

After three or four hours, my friend in the middle fell asleep. Later, I fell asleep. At some point, the driver fell asleep. I heard or sensed an urgency that I needed to wake up immediately. When I woke up, we were going about ninety to one hundred miles an hour. As I looked up, I could not believe what I saw. We were heading right into the back of a mobile home that was being pulled on a trailer. I screamed!

The driver woke up and slammed on the brakes. The truck skidded as we approached the back of the mobile home. I watched in horror as the hood of the El Camino slid under the back of the mobile home. We finally slowed down to the speed of the mobile home, as the back of it came within about one foot of the windshield of the El Camino.

We stopped and pulled over off the road. We got out of the truck just to gather our wits and collect ourselves. Surprisingly, no one needed to change their pants. We should have gotten down on our knees right there and prayed to God for saving our lives with this close call. One more second and we would have been decapitated. But, as invincible young men we thought that it was just luck. Again, I had dodged another bullet.

My Paradigm

It seems that I have needed a tremendous amount of help to stay on the path that God has planned for me. A year or two later while in college, a friend that I played high school football with came to the school I was attending—the University of the Cumberlands. He was into lifting weights and thought he was the meanest, toughest guy around. My friends and I had to continuously listen to him brag. He would tell us how none of us could last in a ring with him for one three-minute round. I guess he was full of young testosterone hormones. I never got into any long arguments with him about it, as it was not important to me. I was just about as strong as he was, much faster, and a better athlete. School and other activities were more important as far as I was concerned.

One night while we were out with friends, we ran into some kids from the local town. There had been some incidents of them jumping college boys and severely assaulting them. My friend, who thought he was the toughest guy around, called them out. One of the guys took him up on it; so a fight was arranged for later that night in a remote area outside of town. Being young men, several of us decided we wanted to watch, as well as several of the local town guys. The fight started between the two.

My friend got his rear-end whipped badly and quickly. He was on the ground, getting kicked, so I grabbed the guy to stop the fight. I actually was happy that he lost the fight, so I would not have to hear him bragging about how tough he was. But, I still needed to stop the fight, before he was seriously injured. As I let the guy go, again a thought or voice told me to duck and get out of the way. One of the town boys had taken off his belt and swung the belt buckle at me. I ducked. The person standing next to me got hit just lateral to his left eye. Another one half inch over and he would have lost his eye.

I took him to the emergency room; he needed more than dozen stitches to close the wound. It was supposed to have been me. Maybe I would have lost an eye. My dream, or more correctly, God's plan for me being an ophthalmologist would have ended. I dodged another bullet. I guess I may be getting good at dodging bullets or my guardian angel has to work overtime.

On three occasions within three or four years, I had very narrow escapes with death or significant injury that would have ended my career as an eye surgeon. A voice or thought came into my mind and saved me on those occasions—ten minutes after listening to the voice or thought on the first occasion and a second on the next two occasions. Each of those times, I brushed off what had happened. I never thought that maybe God had spoken to me or put those thoughts in my mind. Maybe it was because of my age or maybe it was because of a macho male teenage attitude that says I am in charge and invincible. At that time, my paradigm or life was not centered on God, as much as it should have been. We think we are planning and in control of our lives, but God directs our steps!

Many years later, I realized that God must have had other things he wanted me to do. He saved my life. He had a career planned for me. Now that I am a more mature Christian and have become interested in paradigms, I realize that He intervened in my life. There are several other instances that I could tell as well, but those are not as dramatic. These are just three dramatic instances where God saved me.

You may have experienced similar events, where you know that God intervened in your life. There may be many more that you or I may not realize, due to not perceiving that God was working. Maybe you forgot your keys and had to take time to search for them. Therefore, you were not involved in a car accident that would have occurred. We do not always know about all the times that God has helped us follow the plan that He designed for us. Our paradigms may not be tuned into recognizing His work in our lives.

One of the main reasons for writing this book is to show people how to change their paradigms to a more God-centered paradigm and be able to perceive God in their life. You will have a better connection to God. You will be able to see things differently. You will be better at tuning your life or paradigm into God's wavelength or plan for you.

I have prayed and thanked God for the things that He has done for me in my life. I have tried to follow His guidance in pursuing my career. I have thanked Him many times for the times that He saved my life and kept me safe. He protected me from an injury that would have prevented me from being an ophthalmologist.

I have been so blessed to have had the privilege of taking care of my patient's eyes all these years. The smile on their faces when I have restored their vision or have saved their vision is a true blessing. To be so fortunate to have the opportunity to learn so much about the human body that God created has been a real blessing. God's plan for me has been amazing. But, I guess I needed a lot of help getting to where I am today.

Since age seven, I have felt safe and have perceived the presence of the Holy Spirit. Just like most of us, I am very busy. Many times, I have taken my life for granted. I tended not to notice the presence of God or the presence of the Holy Spirit. We tend to look or reach out for God in times of need, facing an issue that you need help with, when worried, in times of stress (such as when I was working in the emergency room or in surgery), or just needing help.

Maybe you can think back on times when you did not understand or realize that God saved your life—that he was working in your life. As you saw in the first chapter everything that you see, perceive, or think you understand may not be what you originally thought. It could be absolutely and totally incorrect. Looking at life with a different paradigm can change the way you see, discern, and react to each thing in life.

Your paradigm is the essence of who you are and your personality. All of us should strive to have our paradigms centered on the love of our Father and Creator. My hope is that after you read this book, you will see God in a more real and significant way. Each day you should take the time to notice how God is intimately involved in the world He created.

**Think about your paradigm
and make changes according
to God's plan for you.
What is your paradigm?**

Chapter 3
Looking Inside Your Brain

1 Corinthians 2:16 NLT

*For, "Who can know the Lord's thoughts?
Who knows enough to teach him?"
But we understand these things,
for we have the mind of Christ.*

Our brain is an amazing creation of God. We are able to think like God in a very small way. In this chapter you are going to learn about your brain. To get a better understanding on how we perceive, understand, observe, and form paradigms, we need to delve into how the brain functions and its anatomy. I will try not to get too technical, but I think that having some background information will be helpful.

The brain is an amazing organ. It is the center, hub, or processor of our nervous system. The word *brain* first appeared in 1,700 B.C. by an unknown Egyptian surgeon. The brain is about the size of a cantaloupe and weighs about three pounds. It is made up of about eighty percent water and the brain is composed of sixty percent fat or lipid. This is not the fat you generally think about, since there are no fat cells in the brain. The fat or lipid in the brain is a major component of the layer that surrounds the axon of the brain cells or neurons as an electrical insulator. It is difficult to know for sure, but there are hundreds or possibly more than a thousand miles of blood vessels in the brain.

The brain is located in the head of all animals, near the location of the five senses: vision, hearing, taste, smell, and sensation. The brain is housed in the skull, which is a bony structure for protection. Twenty percent of the body's total oxygen supply is used to keep the brain functioning. The volume of blood that flows through the brain per minute is about three cans of soda. If your brain loses its blood supply for more than eight seconds or so, you will lose consciousness. The brain can live for only about six minutes without oxygen.

The brain generates up to twenty-five watts of power—your brain could light a twenty-five-watt light bulb! The brain holds about five times the information contained in the Encyclopedia or may have up to one hundred terabytes of information. The brain may perform as many as one hundred trillion calculations per second. The brain does not sense pain, as there are no pain fibers in the brain itself. It is also interesting how the brain is configured. The left side of the brain controls the right side of the body and vice versa.

The brain takes longer than any other organ to develop. Your brain matures around the age of twenty-five. At age three the brain has developed the most neurons and connections and by age eleven the brain starts to prune unused connections. The brain is mostly comprised of two types of cells called neurons and glial cells. The neurons are the brain cells that we use to think. There are one hundred billion neurons in the brain with one quadrillion synapses or connections. They send signals from one neuron to another neuron or to target cells throughout the body. The diameter of a neuron is four microns thick. You could fit thirty thousand neurons on the head of a pin!

The axon carries the signal from the nucleus to the synapse. The axon can transmit signals at a speed of up to two hundred twenty-five miles an hour. We have over one hundred thousand miles of myelinated axons in the brain. The glial cells provide structural support, framework or guidance for development, metabolic support, and insulation.

A neuron in many ways is like other cells in the body. They have similar structures that make up a typical cell. Neurons are different in that they are designed to transmit information from one cell to the next cell. There are three different types of neurons. Sensory neurons carry information from a sensory receptor in the body to the brain. Motor neurons transmit signals to the muscles of the body. Interneurons communicate between other neurons. The neuron cell is composed of three basic parts: the cell body, the axon, and the dendrite.

The cell body houses the nucleus and the cell's DNA. The dendrites look like the branches of a tree which receive information from other neurons. The axon of the neuron transmits information to other cells. The junction between cells is called a synapse. This interface is where the information from one cell is transferred to another. There are chemical and electrical synapses. The electrical synapses are much faster than the chemical synapses. Electrical synapses are involved with certain responses in the body such as the fight or flight response.

The chemicals that are released into the synapse are called neurotransmitters. Neurotransmitters may be excitatory or inhibitory in function, depending on what the neuron is designed to do. You have heard of some of the chemical names in the brain such as serotonin and dopamine. When a neuron is stimulated, it causes a sudden change in its electrical polarity which travels down the axon, where it may stimulate thousands of other neurons or cells. There may be more than one hundred thousand chemical reactions per second occurring in the brain.

Neuron Cell

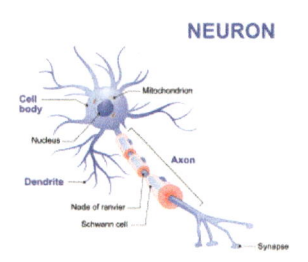

The communication between cells is a central functional component of the brain, which occurs by the synapses of the neurons. There are many different types of synapses. Some excite, some inhibit, and some cause chemical reactions in target cells—like making a muscle contract. The speed at which the axons transmit these signals can be up to one hundred yards a second. Each one of these through all its dendrites may connect to as many as ten thousand other neurons. With all these connections, there may be as many as one hundred trillion connections. Ninety percent of the neurons are located in the cerebral cortex.

The outer region of the cerebral cortex (which is two to four millimeters thick) contains between twenty-two to twenty-five billion neurons. These neurons are capable of performing fifty to sixty million petaflops. A petaflop equals one quadrillion calculations per second. This is on par with the fastest computers in the world. The DNA in the brain and body is a fine spirally coiled thread in the nucleus of the cell body. When stretched out it is six feet long. If you connected all the stands of the DNA in the brain, it would stretch to the sun and nearly half the way back to earth. The brain is a pretty amazing organ that God created.

THE HUMAN BRAIN

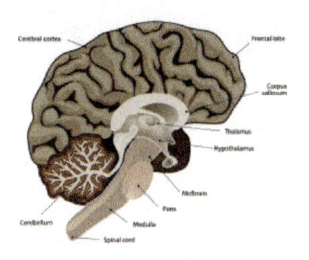

If you are not interested in learning about the specific parts of the brain and their function, skip over to page 67. There I give a short overview.

There are four major components of the central nervous system: spinal cord, brainstem (hindbrain), midbrain (location of portions of the limbic system), and forebrain (cerebral hemispheres). There is also the cerebellum which fine tunes, controls, and regulates the motor function in our bodies. The parts of the brain below the cerebral hemispheres are similar in all animals. Our large cerebral hemispheres and their functions are what make humans different from other animals. As we go up the central nervous system from the spinal cord to the top of the brain where the two cerebral hemispheres are located, there is an increase in the complexity of brain function.

Brainstem or Hindbrain

The brainstem is located at the base of the brain, which is just above the spinal cord. It is responsible for things that are automatic or basic. We don't have to think about them. They are the simple functions of life. The functions that are derived from here are: heart rate, digestion, breathing, eating, drinking, sleeping, eye movements, hearing, and some body movements. This system is similar in all vertebrate animals, as these are the basic functions of living.

The Limbic System or Midbrain

The next level up is an area referred to as the limbic system. The limbic system is an extremely complex set of structures, just underneath the cerebral hemispheres. The limbic system is not a distinct structure, but is composed of several parts of the brain. There is not a consensus on what is included in the limbic system. We are still learning and have a long way to go to understand exactly how the brain and all its parts work. I will go over some of the major structures and functions of the limbic system. Some of the major structures include: hippocampus, amygdala, hypothalamus, thalamus, cingulate gyrus, and olfactory bulb.

You might think of the limbic system from a Biblical standpoint as the flesh. The limbic system is connected to the flow of epinephrine, behavior, emotion, sexual desire, lust, motivation, smell, fear, instinct, insecurity, selfishness, anger, rage, jealousy, envy, aggression, and long term memory. The prefrontal cortex and the limbic system have numerous connections. This area regulates the sympathetic and parasympathetic nervous systems.

The sympathetic nervous system is involved with the fight or flight response in the body. This system is considered excitatory. The parasympathetic nervous system is involved with resting and digesting. This nervous system is considered inhibitory. The two systems tend to counter each other. The sympathetic is responsible for a quick response, while the parasympathetic is a reducing or dampening response. This is a very simplified version of the two systems as there is overlap of their functions. The endocrine system is regulated here. The endocrine system is a collection of glands in the body that produce a variety of hormones that control or regulate growth and development, metabolism, sexual desires and function, mood, reproduction, sleep, and other body functions.

Hippocampus

The hippocampus controls the levels of corticosteroids in the body. It has a role in understanding spatial relations within our environment. It puts together the where, when, and what of life's experiences. This has a direct influence in your perceptions and development of your paradigm. The hippocampus has a major role in memory and is especially important in our short term memories. This area is affected by central nervous system diseases, such as Alzheimer's.

Hypothalamus

The hypothalamus is involved in the autonomic nervous system, endocrine system, and our behavior. Your sexual behaviors are centered in this area of the brain.

Olfactory Bulb

The olfactory bulb receives sensory signals from the nose for smell. In many animals, this is a very important structure. Many animals survive only because of their ability to smell. In humans, its importance is significantly reduced.

Amygdala

The amygdala has a large number of connections to other parts of the brain. It is the critical area in coordinating our responses to fear, danger, stress, and emotional stimuli. It is directly related to the stimulation of your autonomic responses. Stimulation of the amygdala causes your fight or flight reaction, behavior, arousal, and rage. If this area of the brain is over stimulated, it has dire consequences. When the amygdala is overly stimulated, you may not be able to control your emotions and reactions to things that happen to you. This part of the brain gets you into trouble with society, your physical and mental health, and sin against God. This is one of the major sources of mental disease.

Thalamus

The thalamus is involved in the regulation of sleep and consciousness. It serves as a motor and sensory relay in the brain. The thalamus is also involved in the vision pathway from the eye to the vision center of the brain. It relays signals from sensory neurons in regards to touch or sensation and the perception of your body's position in the environment.

Cingulate Gyrus

The cingulate gyrus is involved with the regulation of our emotions, emotion formation, processing, and learning. It links motivation and behavioral outcomes. It is important in depression and schizophrenia. It processes pain and our reactions to pain. It is related to both pains from a physical painful stimulus (such as a hot stove) and emotional pain related to an event in our lives.

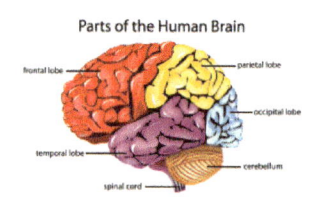

Parts of the Human Brain

Forebrain or Cerebral Hemispheres

The cerebral hemispheres or cerebral cortex is located at the top of the central nervous system. The word cortex means *bark of a tree* and relates to the outer coating of the brain. This is the part of your brain that differentiates you from other animals. Most of the brain functions that I have discussed are common to other animals. Sensory processing from the sensory receptors in your body is one of the main functions of the cerebral cortex. Your ability to think and process information is what makes you different from any other animal.

You may think that teenagers do not have much reasoning ability! As you might have guessed, teenagers are not used to dealing with the new levels of hormones in their bodies. These hormones are stimulating their limbic system at a level they have never experienced before. Therefore, their emotions, perceptions, sex hormones, and their limbic system may be overriding their prefrontal cortex, which is the area of the brain for making decisions.

There are two hemispheres of the cerebral cortex. The hemispheres are connected by the corpus callosum.

There are four different regions of the brain: occipital lobe, parietal lobe, temporal lobe, and frontal lobe.

The Left Hemisphere

Generally speaking, the left hemisphere (or what may be called the dominant hemisphere) deals with the logical and verbal aspects of life. The left hemisphere function is related to logical thinking and linear and/or logical processing. It has to do with language and verbal processing. Attention to detail, analysis of information, and analytic processing are located in the left hemisphere. Academics, the ability to be task oriented, and to formulate goals is the responsibility of the left hemisphere. The entire western civilization and economic development is based on the function of the left hemisphere.

The Right Hemisphere

The right hemisphere (or the non-dominant hemisphere) processes stimuli that are less verbal or logical. The right hemisphere is more art related, poetry, intuitive, and is connected with nonverbal stimuli that we receive from our environment. It analyzes and processes contours, sizes, shapes, and their position or relation to other things or objects. It helps you recognize faces, sounds, tones, and melodies. It gives you your intuition or the ability to read between the lines. Male brains tend to be unilateral in their brain processing, using the left side of their brain. Female brains are efficient at using both sides of their brains. This is one of the major reasons there are problems with communication between the sexes.

Occipital Lobe

The occipital lobe is the vision center of the brain and is located in the back portion of the brain. If you place your hand on the back of your head, that is where the occipital lobe sits. Signals from the retina are sent here to be transformed into what you see. I will go into further detail in the next chapter.

Parietal Lobe

The parietal lobe is located in front and above the occipital lobe. This area can be thought of as the sensation, association, and visual perception center of brain function. It is the location where the brain identifies shapes and then decides what the eye is looking at. It is where most of the processing of perception of what you see in your field of view occurs. The parietal lobe processes sensory information such as touch, two-point discrimination, self-awareness or body-awareness, spatial navigation, cognition, language processing, touch localization, calculation, visuospatial processing or visual perception, and discrimination. The parietal lobe, when stimulated, increases alertness and the ability to relate to other people's feelings and thoughts.

Temporal Lobe

The temporal lobe is located below the parietal lobe and in front of the occipital lobe. The functions of the temporal lobe include sensory processing, vision memories, language comprehension, emotional associations, spatial processing, spirituality, and hearing. The temporal lobe contains the area of the brain that plays a key role in the formation of explicit long term memory modulated by the amygdala. It receives sensory information from the ear for hearing and auditory processing. Areas associated with vision located in the temporal lobe interpret the meaning of what we see.

The temporal lobe establishes object recognition, especially faces and scenes. It deals with object perception and recognition. It processes speech comprehension. It is essential for long term memory storage. There have been studies that have reported that people who suffer seizures involving the temporal lobe have said that they experienced a religious experience.

Frontal Lobe

The frontal lobe is located right behind your forehead. The frontal lobe is extremely complex, with connections to many other parts of the brain. The frontal lobe contains a majority of the dopamine sensitive neurons in the cerebral cortex.

The frontal cortex has to do with being able to project future consequences, choices between good and bad or right and wrong, control of socially unacceptable practices, regulation of behavior, problem solving, determination of differences and similarities to events or things in our environment, organization, concept formation, mental flexibility, personality, judgement, and abstract thinking. The frontal lobe is where imagination, creativity, and originality is born.

The frontal lobe selectively chooses which of the millions of pieces of data or information that it is receiving or reacting to is kept in memory. The rest of the information is discarded. The frontal cortex controls voluntary movements. You decide that you want to look to the left. The frontal cortex sends the message to the midbrain, where the nuclei that control eye muscles are located. The nuclei of the eye muscles then sends the signal to look to the left to the proper eye muscles needed to look to the left. It is the same for walking, playing golf, or tennis.

Prefrontal Cortex

The prefrontal cortex is the front portion of the frontal lobe. Many people consider this area the executive center of the brain. It receives input from many regions of the brain and makes the final decision on perception and actions. All our thoughts, visions, perceptions, and experiences from our environment, eventually come to the prefrontal cortex for final evaluation. It decides what something means, what is important, and what is going to be discarded. In fact, the vast majority of things or data are discarded and not kept in memory. It is responsible for complex thinking and planning, cognitive behavior, moderating social behavior, decision making, and regulating the limbic system especially the amygdala.

The prefrontal cortex is connected to the brainstem and the limbic system. There is a relationship between our levels of arousal and our overall mental status. The prefrontal cortex is paramount in keeping things in balance. You need your prefrontal cortex to keep the amygdala and limbic system under control.

Anterior Cingulate Cortex

The anterior cingulate cortex is located in front of the corpus callosum (the area of connection between the two hemispheres) and next to the prefrontal cortex. It is the critical connection between the prefrontal cortex (our decision making portion of the brain) and the limbic system (portion of the brain related to emotions, sexual arousal, fight or flight responses). It is through this connection that our frontal lobe monitors and tries to regulate the limbic system. It is involved with error detection, emotional regulation, conflict evaluation, moral and ethical evaluation, empathy, strategic planning, focused attention, personality, and participates in developing our paradigms. It is necessary for our empathy and compassion.

I believe it is the primary center of your neurological soul. This is where the battle is between choosing right and wrong—the Holy Spirit urging you not to sin and your limbic system telling you that it is ok to do what feels good at the moment.

Summary of Brain Anatomy

There are four major components of the central nervous system: spinal cord, brainstem, midbrain or limbic system, and cerebral hemispheres.

- The spinal cord carries messages to and from the brain throughout the body.
- The brainstem is responsible for routine body functions, such as breathing, heart rate, and etc.
- The limbic system is responsible for your emotions, such as fear, worry, stress, sex drive, rage. I would consider it the part of the brain that the Bible refers to as your flesh.
- All brains of animals are similar up to this point. The cerebral hemispheres are what distinguishes man from other animals. This is where you think, contemplate, and make decisions.

There is a constant battle in man between the emotions of the limbic system (flesh) and the logical decision making of the cerebral hemispheres. How you live your life depends on how well your prefrontal cortex of your frontal lobe controls your limbic system.

God Circuits in the Brain

Andrew Newburg, M.D. and Mark Waldman are researchers at the University of Pennsylvania's Center for Spirituality and the Mind. Dr. Newburg is the leading authority in the study of a neurological basis for religion. He has written several books. His book called *How God Changes Your Brain* is a great resource. If you would like further information about this subject, read his books.

Curt Thompson, M.D. has written an excellent book called *The Anatomy of the Soul*. Dr. Thompson is a psychiatrist and writes about his experience in his practice and religion.

Timothy Jennings, M.D. wrote the book called *The God-Shaped Brain*. This book is also an excellent resource on the subject of God and your brain.

These are fascinating books about God, religion, and our brains.

Occipital-Parietal Lobe

The occipital-parietal lobe identifies God as an object that exists in the world.

Parietal-Frontal Circuit

The parietal-frontal circuit establishes a relationship between two objects—you and God.

Frontal Lobe

The frontal lobe creates, conceptualizes, and integrates all your ideas about God.

Anterior Cingulate Cortex

This is the part of the brain where I believe that your heart and/or soul is primarily located. You experience love, empathy, and compassion. Your soul decides how you are going to live your life.

Thalamus

The thalamus gives you emotional meaning to your concept and relationship to God. It helps make God seem real. If you engage specific neural circuits, it will allow you to sense or envision a benevolent God, universe, and yourself.

Awareness of the functions of the mind leads to a greater intimacy with God and friends. Awareness is critical in developing a God-centered paradigm.

Temporal Lobe

The temporal lobe allows some people to hear God's voice. As I mentioned earlier, people who have seizures in this area have reported religious experiences.

Occipital Lobe

This helps you envision an anthropomorphic God.

Brain Function and Processing

Today we have various neuroimaging technologies for examining the brain and its function. My wife, Janice, has been in the radiology business for over thirty years. Just like the other fields of medicine, there have been tremendous advances in technology. The brain can be studied with positron-emission tomography (PET scan), functional magnetic resonance imaging (fMRI), and single photon emission computed tomography (SPECT). These systems allow researchers to compare the intensity and location of activity in the different areas of the brain across different circumstances. This could include things such as a person praying, meditating, or looking at various pictures, images, and/or words. We don't think or experience anything without there being a corresponding group of neurons firing that represent that experience.

Until recently, it was felt that your brain was rigid. After you grow and mature, the brain is set. It does not have the ability to grow or change. The old saying that *you cannot teach an old dog new tricks* was considered true. The brain actually has significant plasticity or the ability to change. The brain is constantly working, while we are awake or asleep. It is in a continuous state of flux. Every single second new neurons are being formed. New circuits of neurons are being developed with new axons, and complex networks of dendrites are extending out to other cells. At the same time, neurons that are not being used are being trimmed or pruned.

Another old saying like *you never forget how to ride a bicycle* is true. Many of those neurons are still there. But years later you won't be able to ride it with the same proficiency as you did before— like with no hands. You can gain that proficiency back by practice or stimulating the development of new neurons. You can build new neurons and circuits that have been pruned away. You cannot play golf like Tiger Woods or basketball like Michael Jordan without a lot of practice or repetition to develop neurons for that sport. You also may not have the talent to get to that level either.

A repetition of thought, learning, or physical activity is necessary to improve in any endeavor. In ophthalmology, once a child reaches the age of six or seven their vision is at its optimal level. If they have a lazy eye (crossed eyes) or large difference in being nearsighted or farsighted, they develop amblyopia or loss of vision. You must correct their problem before age six, if they are to obtain good vision. We now know that it is possible to improve the vision later in life with certain vision exercises. Maybe not back to 20/20 vision, but improve the vision a few lines further down the eye chart.

Sometimes when people have cataract surgery with multifocal lenses, they initially have trouble with their vision. They may actually see 20/20, but because the bifocal lens splits the images in the eye into a near image and a distance image, their perception of how they are seeing is different. They have never had vision that works in that manner. Most people will get used to the lenses with time. We call this cortical or neural adaption. The brain learns how use the new vision. The person's brain adjusts to their new vision. There are computer programs that have been developed to help with neural adaption of the vision system and loss of vision from strokes.

The brain is constantly changing. We are learning new things and removing old neurons that are not being used. The plasticity of the brain allows you to change how your brain functions. Dr. Newburg's research at the University of Pennsylvania has demonstrated that God is a part of our conscience. If you contemplate long enough, something astonishing happens in the brain.

The neural functioning of the brain changes. New neurons are made, different circuits are activated, and others become deactivated during this time. New dendrites are formed, new synaptic connections are created, and the brain becomes more sensitive to the subtle realms of experience. Perception or your paradigm alters as you develop a new paradigm. Therefore, your beliefs begin to change, faith has evolved, and God becomes neurologically real.

A Christian brain is different. The brain actually becomes larger and healthier. It is like your spirit in your brain has been dormant waiting for God's Holy Spirit. The Holy Spirit connects to your spirit and new brain functioning occurs. You may have heard, *There is a missing place in your heart that only God can fill.* This missing spot in the heart is in your brain. Your spirit is waiting and only God's spirit can awaken your spirit. The connection of your spirit and the Holy Spirit creates a new brain. According to the Bible, you are *a new creature* or what I call a new paradigm centered on God.

God's Spirit and His love strengthen the anterior cingulate cortex and calm the limbic system. Fear, anxiety, worry, and all the negative emotions are diminished.

1 John 4:18 NLT
Perfect love drives out fear.

The amygdala is not rapidly firing out of control. Your brain is healthier, larger, and more balanced. There are also other health benefits of a God-centered paradigm which I will cover in a later chapter.

The brain is an unbelievable masterpiece. A brain filled with the Holy Spirit is a completed fully functioning brain.

Awareness of your brain's functions is critical to a life full of joy, peace, and love. Your brain is waiting to be fine-tuned to God's wavelength!

Chapter 4
Seeing is Believing (Maybe?)
or
Your Perception

Matthew 6:22

*Your eye is like a lamp that provides light for your body.
When your eye is healthy, your whole body is filled with light.*

Acts 2:17 NLV

*God says, 'In the last days I will send my spirit on all men.
Then your sons and daughters will speak God's Word.
Your young men will see what God has given them to see.
Your old men will dream dreams.*

It appears God is telling you that what you see and observe in your life is extremely important. The way you see, through eyes filled with the Holy Spirit, allows you to perceive things in your life differently from other non-Christian people. What you see, observe, interpret, and perceive can affect the wellness and health of your whole body.

As an ophthalmologist, the eye and our vision system has been my life's work. I have had the privilege of helping many people with their vision—from glasses to surgery. Nearly everything you do in your daily life involves using your vision to complete the task. Obviously people who are blind can live full productive happy lives, but they do have some limitations.

The Bible talks about light—that Jesus is the light unto the world. The Bible also gives a characteristic of light in John.

John 1:5 NLT—*The light shines in darkness and the darkness can never extinguish it.*

Do you know that in a completely dark environment, a single candle can be seen up to thirty miles away? If you can set a candle on a mountain top, so that you can see around the curvature of the earth, you can see it up to thirty miles away. Light is always dominant over darkness—spiritually and physically.

What is *light* that we need to use it in order to see? Light is electromagnetic radiation, which is produced by vibrations of a charged material. There is a very wide spectrum of electromagnetic radiation wavelengths and visible light is only a small portion. Visible light waves have wavelengths between 400 and 700 nanometers. The colors in the rainbow are composed of these wavelengths of light.

A rainbow is caused by dispersion, refraction, and reflection of light in the raindrops. The rainbow is classically described as having seven colors. Rainbows actually are a continuous blend or spectrum of colors. At the distance that we are looking at rainbows, we are unable to see more than seven colors. The colors starting from the outer color to the inner color are red, orange, yellow, green, blue, indigo, and violet. The rainbow forms as the light enters and exits the rain drops, separating the color of visible light. God formed the rainbow as a covenant with earth.

> *Then God told Noah and his sons, "I hereby confirm my covenant with you and your descendants, and with all the animals that were on the boat with you—the birds, the livestock, and all the wild animals—every living creature on earth. Yes, I am confirming my covenant with you. Never again will the flood waters kill all living creatures; never again will a flood*

destroy the earth." Then God said, "I am giving you a sign of my covenant with you and with all living creatures, for all generations to come. I have placed my rainbow in the clouds. It is the sign of my covenant with you and with all the earth. When I send clouds over the earth, the rainbow will appear in the clouds and I will remember my covenant with you and with all living creatures. Never again will the floodwaters destroy all life. When I see the rainbow in the clouds, I will remember the eternal covenant between God and every living creature on earth." Then God said to Noah, "Yes, this rainbow is the sign of the covenant I am confirming with all the creatures on earth."

Genesis 9:8-17 NLT

I know that it could be me and how I think with my paradigm, but was there a rainbow before God confirmed His covenant with a rainbow? Did God change the physics of rain drops, so that when light shined through the rain, the prism effect on light caused the rainbow to develop? I always try to look at things from a different perspective. You never know what you might discover!

God made this world beautiful. His masterful hand is everywhere to be seen. It is amazing how intricate and complicated it is. When we look at this world, we see the simple superficial beauty. Most of us don't take the time to observe the absolutely amazing things God has created.

When I am scuba diving, I always look for a cleaning station. A cleaning station is where a larger fish (such as a grouper) parks itself next to a reef. There is no sign on the reef indicating the location of the cleaning station. The fish just know where it is. God has created every minute detail of the universe. A cleaning station for fish is like us taking our car to the carwash to get it cleaned.

The grouper remains stationary next to the reef. The fish opens its mouth and spreads open its gills. These beautiful cleaner shrimp with clear bodies and internal organs of bright blue and red colors suddenly appear. They have white spots on their clear shells. They swim out to the grouper. Also, small brightly colored cleaner wrasse fish swim out from the reef. They swim and crawl inside the grouper's mouth, around the outside of the fish, and enter the gills of the fish to clean any parasites off the grouper. The grouper never eats these delicious morsels. When they are finished cleaning the grouper, they swim back to the reef. The fish swims away all clean. It is amazing watching this symbiotic relationship.

God has developed this fantastically complex and beautiful world. We all need to take time to look further into His intricate design. Have you ever spent time watching a spider build its web? An architect couldn't build it better. The spider has the brain the size of a poppy seed. But, God has given the spider the ability to make its beautiful symmetrical web. Each day spend a couple minutes observing the vastness and complexity of this world. Doing this will help you understand God in a deeper and more meaningful way.

Why is the sky blue? Many of you may already know, but many of you may find it interesting. The atmosphere is composed mostly of nitrogen and oxygen, along with other gases and water vapor. It is denser near the earth's surface and becomes thinner towards space. Light travels or radiates in waves. Violet light has the shortest wavelength. The blue color of the sky is caused by the particles in the atmosphere which scatter the shorter blue light rays of light. The reds, oranges, and yellow light waves are longer and pass through the atmosphere. The red colors at sunset are due to the fact that the light has to pass through more of the atmosphere because of the angle of the light from the sun. All the blue light has been filtered out. We are left with reds and oranges. The Bible actually talks about the red sky as a sign to be used to predict the weather.

Matthew 16:2-3 NLT

He replied, You know the saying, 'Red sky at night means fair weather tomorrow; red sky in the morning means foul weather all day.'

This is related to the amount of moisture in the atmosphere.

Energy (electron volts, eV)									
10^8	10^6	10^4	10^2	1	10^{-2}	10^{-4}	10^{-6}	10^{-8}	10^{-8}
gamma rays	X-rays		ultraviolet rays	infrared rays		radar	FM TV	short-wave	AM
10^{-14}	10^{-12}	10^{-10}	10^{-8}	10^{-6}	10^{-4}	10^{-2}	1	10^2	10^4

Wavelength (meters, m)

Visible light

400 — 500 — 600 — 700

Wavelength (nanometers, nm)

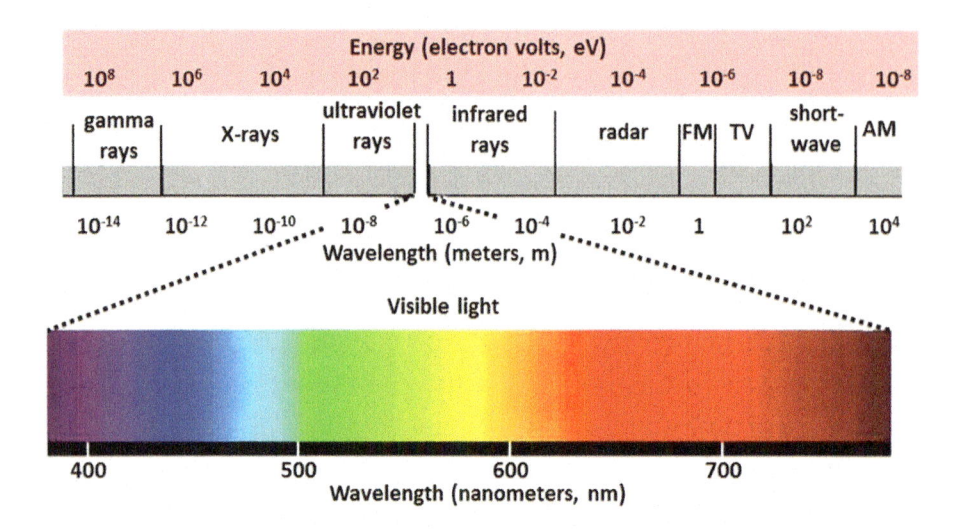

Everyone has heard about lasers. They have been used in ophthalmology since the 1950s. There are now many different lasers used in ophthalmology for treating glaucoma, retinal diseases, vision correction, and during cataract surgery. A laser is composed of a single wavelength of light. Different wavelengths have different properties which are used in medicine, the military, and a large variety of industries. There are lasers that cut with heat and are called *hot lasers*. There are lasers that cut without generating any heat that are called *cold lasers*. The characteristic of a laser depends on the wavelength chosen.

A wavelength for a laser device is chosen based on the task that it is going to be design to perform. They are unbelievably accurate. Many of you have seen the bombs that the military has used in war. You may have watched them on television as the missile is guided through a window in a building. This is accomplished by using a laser for guidance called a YAG laser. Light can be used for many things other than for vision.

Everyone has heard the term *20/20 vision*. I am frequently asked, "What is 20/20 vision?" It was determined that normal clear vision is when a person can see the difference between the letter C versus an O at twenty feet. That gap in the letter C is 1 minute of arc at 20 feet. A person with 20/40 vision is seeing the size of a letter that a person with 20/20 vision can see at 40 feet versus what they are seeing it at 20 feet. There are still other ways of testing vision that are more sensitive than seeing black letters on a white background. One method is called *contrast sensitivity*. Contrast sensitivity is the ability to see a grey letter on a lighter grey background.

When you are born you have the ability to see objects and colors. Babies are born very nearsighted and see clearly at about ten to fifteen inches from their eyes. By age one or two months, they are able to track and move their eyes together. At about two months their color perception improves, as they can now distinguish shades of colors. At four months of age they develop stereopsis or depth perception. At eight months of age their vision has improved to the point that they can recognize a face from across the room. They may not obtain 20/20 vision until around age four. How your eyes and vision system convert light into what you see is an extremely complex matter.

Your body is constantly receiving sensory information from the five senses. Of course, I am biased in that I believe the vision system is more complex and important to our daily lives than our other senses. In humans, vision is the dominant sense. In some animals such as a shark or other predatory animals, the sense of smell is the dominant sense. People fear vision loss more than almost any other medical condition.

More than ninety percent of communications between people is nonverbal. It is not just the words. It is how the words are delivered that influences how another person perceives what is being communicated. A large portion of the brain deals with vision, perception, reaction to what you see, spatial relationship, and other recognition methods. Half of the body's cranial nerves are related to the eye.

The visual system starts when a light stimulus enters the eye. The light is transmitted to the vision center of the brain, which is the occipital lobe in the back of the brain. The visual pathway has to traverse nearly the entire brain to reach the occipital lobe. Nearly every part of the brain contributes to vision, perception, and understanding of what you see.

Vision and perception are vital to your interactions in this world. Your paradigm directly affects how you interpret what you see. In other animals, others senses may be more important such as smell in sharks or other predatory animals.

The eye actually works very much like a camera. There is a front focusing portion of the eye or camera. The image processing portion is in the back of the eye and camera. A camera has a focusing lens in the front part of the camera and the film or now a computer chip in the back of the camera. Light enters the eye traveling through the tear film on the surface of the cornea. The cornea is the clear portion of the eye in front of the iris or color portion of the eye. The cornea begins the focusing of the light through the opening in the iris or pupil. The light is then focused by the lens located behind the pupil onto the retina.

The retina has ten layers, but you will probably remember from school the terms cones and rods in the retina. The cones provide your color vision and fine detail vision. The rods are for night vision and side vision. These are called photoreceptors. The retina is the inside lining of the eye. The central portion of the retina is called the macula. I am sure that you have heard of macular degeneration or know someone with macular degeneration. The macula is responsible for your central clear fine vision that you use for reading, writing, watching TV, driving a car, etc. When you look directly at an object, you are focusing on that object with your macula. You cannot read anything with your side-vision. As you age, the cells in the macula can degenerate causing loss of vision.

If you or a relative have macular degeneration, there are some things you should do or follow. You should not smoke, protect your eyes from the sun, take a supplement containing the AREDS formula, and follow the diet discussed later in the book. The AREDS study was a very large study conducted across the United States over five years.

It showed that you could decrease the rate at which your macular degeneration progressed by up to forty percent by taking the AREDS formula supplement.

Now let's get back to how you see. The light that enters the eye stimulates the photoreceptors. The photoreceptors convert the light into electrochemical signals. The signal travels to the optic nerve which is an extension of the brain. The optic nerve transmits the signal through the thalamus. The signal travels from the thalamus to the occipital lobes in the back portion of the brain. As light passes through the pupil, it crosses over to the opposite side of the retina. For instance, the light that enters the eye from the right passes through the pupil and lands on the opposite side of the retina. The same happens with light from above and lands on the bottom of the retina. So your eye actually receives the image backwards and upside down. As the stimulus progresses through the vision pathway to the vision center in the brain, the nerve fibers reorient themselves so that you see correctly.

The optic nerves meet in the brain just behind nose in the optic chiasm. The nerves from the nasal halves of both retinas cross over to the vision pathway on the other side of the brain. This cross over of fibers results in your right occipital lobe seeing the left half of your vision in each eye and the left occipital lobe seeing the right half of your vision. The brain then has to bring all this information from each side of the brain to an image that we can see and use.

The brain also has to coordinate the movement of each eye together, so that you will not see double. This is called fusion. Eye movements are controlled in the midbrain, which is a lower order of function. Most animals need to use their eyes together. There are exceptions, such as certain lizards and insects. Scanning across a line while you are reading is controlled by the parietal lobe of the brain. As you can see the vision system is very complicated.

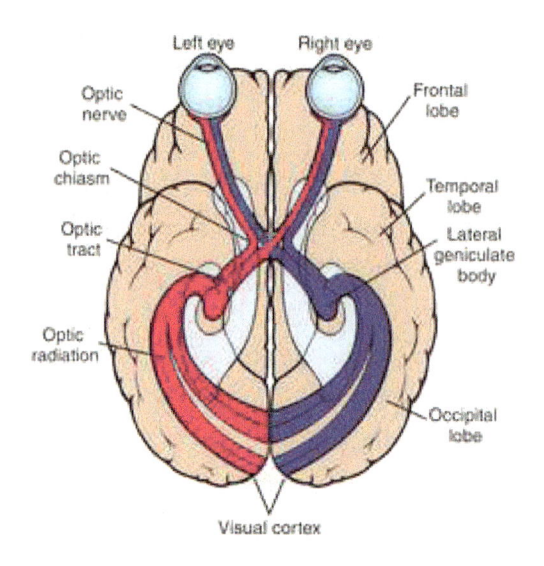

Diagram labels: Left eye, Right eye, Optic nerve, Optic chiasm, Optic tract, Optic radiation, Frontal lobe, Temporal lobe, Lateral geniculate body, Occipital lobe, Visual cortex

Now that the light stimulus has reached the visual cortex in the occipital, the brain is going to start forming the image that the eye just received. The visual cortex is now aligned with what you see in your field of vision. The brain works a little like a computer that uses 0s and 1s. The brain sees by off and on patches. These are called *Gabor patches*. The light stimulus first goes to the primary visual cortex, which primarily deals with basic features such as size, shape, edges, lines of orientation, topography, magnification, and movement or motion. The light or visual stimulus is then transmitted to the secondary visual cortex.

The secondary visual cortex does more refining of our vision into more complex forms. Here we are going from what a child would draw as match stick pictures to where the brain is starting to develop a 3-D, 4K, or Technicolor picture. From the secondary visual cortex there are two main pathways. One is to the neighboring parietal lobe and the other is to the temporal lobe. The parietal lobe processes information relating to location of objects in space or orientation in space. This helps us react in a specific way. We are able to locate an image, catch an object, move our eyes to an object, or turn toward the object.

Seeing is Believing (Maybe?) or Your Perception

The temporal lobe is important in recognizing what the image is. It is amazing, but it appears that there may be specific neurons for a particular image or face. The neuron will only fire if you are looking at the President, movie star, or family member.

What about the colors we see in our vision? Our color vision is based on the trichromatic theory. The primary colors are blue, red, and green. All other colors are derived from a combination of these three colors. Humans can perceive up to ten million shades of color. There are people who are color blind and unable to see colors well. Eight percent of men and one half percent of women are color blind. So eight percent of men have a good reason why they put on clothes that don't match!

There is also the important function called depth perception. You need the ability to judge distances, such as when you are driving a car. You have to have good vision in both eyes in order to have depth perception. You need vision from two different directions to triangulate a distance.

I don't want to get too bogged down in this scientific information about our vision, but I think it is important to know some of the facts. I wanted to give you an idea of how complex our vision system is. Many parts of the brain are involved with what you see. Here is a small partial list of some of the vision functions that are going on in your brain in order for you to see: space perception, relative size, position, familiar size, haze or aerial perspective, linear perspective, vanishing point, anamorphic projection, attention, selective attention, visual search, feature search, guided search, scene guidance, and many more.

As the brain is assimilating all this information about what you are looking at, the brain needs to come to a final conclusion about it. Now that all that information from what you are looking at has tabulated from all the different parts of the brain, this data is then transmitted to the prefrontal cortex. The prefrontal cortex evaluates all the information and then makes a decision about what you believe you are seeing. When you add all this visual information together it leads to what we call perception.

What is Perception?

Perception is the identification, organization, interpretation, and processing of data or information in order to understand our environment. Visual perception is the ability to interpret what you see in your environment. Everything that you receive from your sensory system contributes to how you perceive everything in your world. All five of the senses contribute to your perception.

The next step is to understand how you process that information, which is totally dictated by your individual paradigm. Finally, what decisions do you make based on this processed information.

Let's look at some other definitions of perception. Perception means the ability to see, hear, or become aware of something through using your senses. It is a way of regarding, understanding, or interpreting something or a mental impression. Another definition is intuitive understanding or insight. Perception is the neurophysiological process including memory by which an organism becomes aware of and interprets external stimuli. Perception is the organization, identification, and interpretation of sensory signals from all your sensory receptors in your body brought to your mind through the central nervous system. Some synonyms for perception may give you a deeper understanding of perception. These are awareness, consciousness, feeling, sensation, apprehending, realizing, recognition, discernment, observation, insight, grasp, and comprehension.

Here are some famous quotes about perception.

There are things known and there are things unknown, and in between are the doors of perception.

— Aldous Huxley

Perception is reality. If you are perceived to be something, you might as well be it because that's the truth in people's minds.

— Steve Young

Seeing is Believing (Maybe?) or Your Perception

One has not only an ability to perceive the world but an ability to alter one's perception of it; more simply, one can change things by the manner in which one looks at them.

— Tom Robbins

What you see and hear depends a good deal on where you are standing; it also depends on what sort of person you are.

— C.S. Lewis

The eye sees only what the mind is prepared to comprehend.

— Robertson Davies

The brain forms and develops the world that you are looking at from two different and separate images from each eye or retina. Perception is a very complex function; most of the time you are unaware of the process. Your brain smooths out your perception and vision as the input is incomplete and variable. You do not see the blood flowing through your retina, even though it is there. (There are ways to actually see the blood flow, but it might drive you crazy until your brain smooths it away.) You don't see the blind spot in your vision, as you have no vision where the optic nerve exits from the eye. The brain smooths over that area, as it extrapolates and fills in the vision for that area of your sight. The major problem in perception is what you see is not just the translation of the light that the retina receives. Your perception is influenced by many other factors as you will see as I go through how perception occurs.

Hermann von Helmholtz is thought of as the first to study perception in modern times. He thought that the human eye was optically poor. Compared to a hawk or eagle, he is correct. He concluded that vision could only be the result of some form of unconscious inferences and a matter of making assumptions and conclusions from incomplete data based on previous experiences (or paradigm, my insertion).

Perception can be divided into two basic processes. The first process involves transforming low-level information from the sensory receptors. The second process involves the connection of a person's prior experience, concepts, knowledge, expectations, attention, and selective mechanisms.

This gets us to the crux of paradigms. Perceptions are based on experience, motivational state, and emotional state. Ambiguity and the lack of complete information can be exploited by human technology in things such as the design of camouflage or in the images you saw in the first chapter. Some of the components of perception are constancy, grouping, contrast effects, experience, motivation, and expectation.

Constancy is the ability to recognize an object from a variety of angles. You can recognize someone from behind or the side based on constancy.

Grouping is a set of principles proposed by Gestalt psychologists to explain how humans perceive objects based on patterns. This is called the Gestalt Laws of Organization. The factors involved are proximity, similarity, closure, symmetry, common motion, continuity, regular pattern, and past experience. I am not going to go into each one, but you can grasp the meaning of each factor.

An example of contrast effects is that lukewarm water can be perceived as hot or cold. It all depends on if the hand was in hot or cold water before being placed in the lukewarm water.

As stated before, experience is a major influence on perception. Expectation contributes to perception. When making rounds in a hospital, I never pay attention to the announcements; but I immediately recognize my name if paged.

Motivation influences your perception. What you see in a game is tremendously affected by your connection to a team. A particular call in the game will appear a certain way, because your team is playing.

Through experience and training the brain is able to make finer distinctions, better awareness, and understanding. Your paradigm can continue to change and improve, in whatever you endeavor to accomplish or understand. Your vision is the dominant sense that you use for perception, but the other senses are important as well. As an ophthalmologist I am obviously biased about vision. The other senses do contribute to your perception and can add to the image or scene that you are looking at.

If there is a strong sense of smell associated with an image, it becomes a much stronger memory. More than fifty percent of the brain is used for processing sensory information from your sensory receptors. Your body is full of sensory receptors; you are constantly processing sensory information. It is just that most of it is done subconsciously. You are aware of it only when you decide to pay attention to something you may sense as special, or if there is an unusual strong sensation. Your five senses of vision, hearing, touch, taste, and smell are your connection to the world that you live in. God gave you this sensory system for you to use in your daily life, but it is also to be used as a connection to Him.

You hear because your ear detects vibrations. The ear can hear vibrations between 20 Hz and 20,000 Hz. Speech perception is the process in which the sound of language is heard, interpreted, and understood. The sound of a word can vary dramatically according to the words around it, the speed or tempo of the speech, the appearance and mannerisms of the person giving the speech, and accent of the speaker.

Touch perception is the process of recognizing an object by simply touching it. The surface of the skin can perceive texture, edges, and curvatures which is called proprioception.

Taste is obviously the ability to perceive the flavor of what you are eating. There are approximately ten thousand taste buds with up to one hundred fifty taste receptors cells on each taste bud on the tongue. There are now five recognized tastes. These are salt, bitter, sweet, sour, and now umami. A new taste has been discovered which is due to a fatty acid in fat.

Attention is a vital aspect of perception, because you are unable to process all the input from your senses, especially vision. As I stated before, you discard the vast majority of the sensory information that your brain processes. When you search for something, you typically look for a target item in space among a vast number of things in what you are looking at. Perceptions can be ambiguous. Perceptions change as you age and gain experience. Many times what you think you see is not accurate. The brain fills in the gaps in your perception which is determined by each person's paradigm.

You are guided by your knowledge of known objects or your paradigm. Some perceptions involve selective and non-selective processing. You are able to remember thousands of images after only a second or two of exposure to the images. But in contrast, you can miss large changes in scenes, if these changes do not markedly alter the meaning of the scene.

One interesting example of this is a study where a person is giving directions to someone on the sidewalk. During the instructions two men carrying a large picture walk between the two people. There is a person following behind the picture and they take the place of the person receiving the instructions. The original person receiving the instructions leaves walking behind the picture. A large percentage of people continue giving the instructions after the picture has passed. They never notice that they are speaking to a different individual. It is amazing how our minds work.

What is reality?

The talk of perception needs to be followed by a discussion of reality. According to Dictionary.com, reality is:
- The state or quality of being real
- Resemblance to what is real
- A real thing
- Something that exits independently of ideas concerning it

- Something that exists independently of all other things and from which all other things derive
- Something that constitutes a real or actual thing, as distinguished from something that is merely apparent

Your perception of things is related to your paradigm and may be different from reality.

Just like the discussion of paradigms in the first chapter, you may not see or observe correctly a factual event. Just because you see something, you assume that it is real. My fishing partners thought there were no tarpon around until we caught one, because they could not see the fish. Your personal perceptions can actually cloud or hide reality. Some people feel that reality is not absolute, but is in the eye of the beholder. The implication is that reality itself can change from person to person based on their perceptions.

You can see from the definition that reality is independent of ideas, beliefs, or thoughts. Reality is fact or true. Reality is a law or principle. It is important to differentiate between a principle and an opinion. There are people who get into long discussions about reality from different theories. I am not going to get into that discussion. Let's make it simple.

God created this universe with specific laws and principles. That is reality as God has created it in this world. You are unable to have any knowledge other than what is present in this world. Laws and principles can only be discovered, not created, by man. A major stumbling block to perceiving reality is a person's paradigm. You need to be open to a new paradigm in order to see reality at times. As a pursuer of truth, you need to be willing to give up your biases. God's laws and principles are true, factual, and never change.

The vision system, as I said earlier, is extremely complex. There are many areas of the brain that contribute to the final vision product. Different areas of the brain have a specific function, such as face recognition, motion, and assimilating all the fine details of what we are looking at. The brain compares and combines what we have seen in the past and compares it to the current image. Sometimes the brain fills in gaps in our vision from past experience. This is where your paradigm affects your perception. You cannot process everything you see at once. Our brain, as fantastically as it was designed by God, doesn't have the capacity.

What you choose to process in your mind depends on your individual paradigm. The prefrontal cortex makes assumptions based on your paradigm and that can alter your perception of what you see. This perception is your reality, which you hope is actual and true. This then effects how you react to what you see. You may not react appropriately due to your perception. You may totally miss what your eyes are seeing. Remember the playing cards and the dual images in the chapter on paradigms. Unfortunately, many people have been executed or are in jail due to poor perception or recognition due to the paradigm of a particular witness.

You need to take time to train your brain to understand and perceive things that you may not have understood or perceived before. You can use your perceptions in a more productive manner. It is good to look past what may seem obvious, to find a better answer or to understand something from a different perspective. As the old adage goes, *thinking outside the box.*

Brain Plasticity

Depending on how far you want to go with training your brain, you could even improve the quality of your vision. The FBI is an expert in training its people's observation skills. There is a software program by Revital Vision that uses a Gabor patch system to train the brain to see better. You can also protect your vision by eating plenty of dark green vegetables and oily fish. Smoking causes cataracts to develop at a younger age and is a risk factor for developing macular degeneration. Sun exposure or UV light can also cause cataracts to develop at a younger age. There is some evidence that UV exposure is related to macular degeneration. Always wear sunglasses (and a hat is a good idea, as well) anytime you are outdoors.

As Helen Keller once said, "The thing that is worse than being blind is having sight but no vision."

As you saw in the first chapter, your eye or perception can be fooled or wrong depending on your paradigm. As an ophthalmologist, I believe that vision is paramount. You will never be able see into or understand God's spiritual realm, but God does come to us in this world. God created everything in your body, so that your eyes would be able to see and enjoy this world that He has created. You will be able to be nearer to Him by recognizing Him in this world and your life. I am not just talking about 20/20 vision, but true real vision or perception.

True perception in this world needs to be based on God's vision of His creation. Such as, God looks at a person from the inside out. We tend to look from the outside in. We are sinners and have rejected Him time and time again. But, He still looks at us with His eyes of love.

Go to YouTube and search God Whispers yt.wmv. This is a great video about seeing and perceiving God in this world. Also search for God's Beautiful Creation, Awesome Scenery on YouTube. *God is everywhere.*

**<center>Learn to look and perceive this world
with God-centered paradigm eyes of faith
for true perception!</center>**

Chapter 5
Health Benefits of a God-Centered Paradigm

1 Kings 3:14 NLV

And if you walk in My ways and keep My laws and Word as your father David did, I will allow you to live a long time.

How can your paradigm affect your health?

When I took a course on paradigms, the company gave many examples of paradigms and how they affect us. One example they gave was a study they did on a NFL football team. They got permission to do this study from one of the teams. This was completed during training camp before the season began. They divided the team in half. The first group was brought into a room one player at a time. They were told how great they looked, how strong they looked, asked how much weight they were lifting, and so forth. Although they measured many different parts of their bodies, I will report only on their chest measurements. They asked the players to inhale completely, and then they measured their chest size. The next group came into the room. They asked them if they were feeling well, said they looked tired, asked was training camp going OK, and so forth. They asked them to inhale completely and they measured their chest size.

Two weeks later they reversed what they said to the two groups of players. The difference in maximum chest size between being told how great they looked versus how bad they looked averaged 1 ½ inches. So, just being told how you look or how you may be feeling can make a significant measurable difference in you physically.

In sports, you hear about how a particular athlete is aware of the whole playing field. What is unique about them? They seem to have an ability that other players don't appear to have. You see other athletes that never succeed, even though they have great talent. The stress related to playing a sport is handled differently between each athlete. Some are unable to handle and control their limbic systems during the game. They may suffer from loss of side vision or tunnel vision. They play like they have blinders on. The stress and anxiety of the game doesn't allow their vision or their muscles to perform properly.

You have heard the term *choke*. I remember a game in high school where a teammate of mine choked. It was near the end of the game and the score was tied. He was fouled and we needed him to make the free throws. Everyone was watching him and I could see that the pressure of the situation was getting to him. I could see the look in his eyes and his body posture that it was not going to be good. He shot the free throw and it was five feet short of getting to the goal! I have never seen someone choke that badly. His muscles tightened so much that he had no strength.

Other players are able or even enjoy everything associated with playing the game. They are described as a field general. They see everything that is happening on the court or playing field. The television commentators state that the player has command of the whole playing field.

Not controlling your emotions and limbic portion of the brain causes decreased activity in other important portions of the brain. Under stress people will not make good rational decisions using their prefrontal cortex or perform physically well. Long term stress does do damage to your health.

In *JAMA Psychiatry*, February 2014 (JAMA is the Journal of American Medical Association) an article titled *Neuroanatomical*

Correlates of Religiosity and Spirituality reports that people who believe in the importance of religion or spirituality have thicker brain cortexes. It is believed that this may confer resilience to the development of depressive illness in individuals at high familial risk for major depression.

As you read through this chapter, you will see that having a God-centered paradigm will create less stress, worry, anger, fear, and anxiety in your life and/or you will handle these in a better way. Your brain and body functions perform in a more natural way.

Having a God-centered paradigm leads to better health. At first you may think, how is this possible? One of the major reasons for poor health in this modern world is stress and anxiety. There are studies that show up to 75% of diseases are related to stress and anxiety. There are studies that show up to 75% of deaths are related to life-style habits of smoking, over eating and/or overweight, and alcohol consumption. Other major contributors for poor health are worry, fear, and anger which lead to the variety of different anxiety related diseases. Our lives today are non-stop, with everyone trying to succeed in whatever their life is involved in.

Whether it is work, raising kids, sports, maintaining a household, or others things that you place importance on, how you handle the stress and anxiety in your life determines the quality of your health. A lot of the time these things occupy or sometimes control your life. If you are not careful this can lead to an abnormal amount of stress. Your body is made to handle a normal amount of stress; but if the stress gets out of control, it leads to damage to your body.

Unfortunately, many people run the rat race of life and they suffer because of this. They worry about everything and everyone. Many people are fearful that they won't be successful, everything has to be perfect, and they even worry about what might happen. What if this doesn't work or if this happens, then what are you going to do?

You get cut off in traffic and become very angry at the person who cut in front of you. You scream and yell at that person. Your blood pressure shoots up, heart rate increases, and your limbic system which has not been turned on is now releasing all the chemicals to rev up your body. The person you are upset about may not even pay attention to what you are doing or be aware of what they did. You have activated the fight or flight response of the body which begins in the amygdala and other portions of the limbic system. The sympathetic nervous system is stimulated releasing a cascade of hormones such as catecholamine (epinephrine and norepinephrine), cortisol, and other hormones. The result of stimulating your limbic system is a significant change in the functioning of your body.

Here is a list of some of the changes that occur in your body;

- Increased blood pressure
- Increased heart rate
- Increased breathing
- Increased blood sugar
- Constriction of blood vessels in many parts of the body
- Suppression of the immune system
- Increased boost of energy
- Muscles in the body are prepared for intense usage
- Flushing of the skin
- Sphincters in the body tighten
- Shaking
- Loss of hearing
- Dilation of the pupils
- Tunnel vision

You probably had no idea what the body is doing under these conditions. Stimulating the amygdala and limbic system constantly has long deleterious effects on the body.

All this stress, worry, anger, fear, anxiety, and hyperactive body functions cause the body to release free radicals in your body. Your body is designed to handle a normal number of free radicals. You release free radicals constantly as the cells in your body do their jobs. The free radicals are a byproduct of the cells working—just like the exhaust from a car engine running. Other causes for the release of free radicals are poor diet, pollution, toxins, cigarette smoke, certain drugs, pesticides, and poor sleep habits.

What is a *free radical*? A free radical is a molecule that has an unpaired electron on its outer shell. These molecules or atoms are unstable with their unpaired electron on their surface. They need to add an electron or lose their unpaired electron, so that they will become stable. Damage to other cells occur as the free radical removes an electron from a nearby cell. Now that cell is damaged, and it tries to do the same thing. This starts a chain reaction in the body. As you live your life with high levels of stress and anxiety, you produce more free radicals.

Another term similar to free radical damage is *oxidative damage*. Oxidative stress is the imbalance between the production of free radicals and the ability of the body to neutralize the free radicals. Oxidative stress damages protein and DNA in the body. Oxidative stress damages proteins in the body which affects the activity of enzymes, receptors, and membrane transport. This leads to aging in the body. DNA and RNA are susceptible to oxidative damage. Oxidative damage and free radical damage has been linked to diseases such as cancer, Alzheimer's disease, other similar neurologic diseases, atherosclerosis, diabetes, arthritis, increased aging, stroke, heart disease, depression, vasculitis, gastric ulcers, Parkinson's disease, and anxiety disorders.

The brain is especially vulnerable to oxidative stress and free radical production. The brain uses 20% of the body's oxygen. The brain is fat or lipid rich which makes it vulnerable to oxidation and has limited antioxidant protection. Nervous system diseases such as neurodegenerative diseases and neuropsychiatric diseases are associated with free radicals and oxidative stress. Free radicals cause progressive damage to the cells in the body that accumulate as we age.

An antioxidant is a molecule that is very stable and able to donate an electron to a rampaging free radical. This stabilizes or neutralizes the free radical. The antioxidants decrease cellular damage through their free radical scavenging properties. Cells in the body are protected against free radicals and oxidative stress by antioxidant enzymes. The body produces molecules that are antioxidant. It is when there are more free radicals than the body can manage that damage occurs.

In the beginning the major known antioxidants that we could get from outside the body were vitamin C, vitamin E, and B-carotene. Other antioxidants are melatonin, lutein, lycopene, selenium, vitamin A, and Zinc. You can get these in a diet of fruits and vegetables or through taking supplements. There is some controversy in medicine about whether taking supplements or vitamins is beneficial. I can tell you that from an ophthalmologist's point of view, we do have studies in macular degeneration that show taking an AREDS 2 vitamin formula can significantly reduce the progression of dry macular degeneration.

Another great source for getting healthy nutrients is from herbs and spices. Turmeric is my favorite spice that I like to use. It has many beneficial properties. Others are onions, garlic, ginger, curries, cloves, mustard, red chilies, fenugreek, curry leaf, and Indian medicinal plants. Phytochemicals or phytonutrients are found in good concentrations in any vegetable with bright or dark colors. There is now a big industry of growing crops for health, rather than just for food. Kale is now readily available in the grocery store. It is one of the best vegetables that you can eat, as far as nutritional value is concerned. These are now called functional foods. Though it is very controversial, the development of genetically engineered plants can produce vegetables with more nutritional value, such as tomatoes with up to three times the lycopene. There are many polyphenolic compounds that are healthy. You can find a list at the following site if you are interested. Table 3 JAPI VOL 52 October 2004 www.japi.org .

Decreasing your free radicals is an important step in being healthy and living a long life.

Chronically over stimulating your limbic system can increase the incidence of type 2 diabetes, obesity, increased cholesterol and triglycerides, ulcers, inflammatory diseases, heart attack, stroke, decreased immune system and increased infection, pain, sleep disorders, chronic fatigue syndrome, and fibromyalgia.

Recently there have been studies that link free radicals and oxidative stress to the development of anxiety. Anxiety is a normal response to a potential threat, fear of a particular event (speaking in front of a large group of people), or before participating in a sporting event. When the anxiety is beyond what would be an appropriate level, it is severe, and/or constant, it becomes a disease. Anxiety causes our brains to function abnormally. Anxiety disorders may affect as much as 30% of the American population. It is one of the most common psychiatric diseases in America. Anxiety can cause a variety of disorders such as panic attacks, obsessive-compulsive disorders, depression, and other psychiatric diseases.

Anger is another negative emotion that can affect your health. Chronic anger can increase the risk of having a heart attack or stroke. During the two hours after an anger outburst, your chance of having a heart attack or stroke doubles. Anger will make your anxiety worse. It decreases your lung capacity and shortens your life.

In order to make good wise decisions in life, you need to stop stimulating your amygdala and limbic system. When the limbic system is firing at a high rate, your prefrontal cortex is not functioning properly. You are unable to make logical decisions under stress and anxiety.

All these negative emotions are harmful to your health. Later in the book I will go over ways to change your paradigm, but for now here are some Bible verses—as God is the ultimate healer.

John 14:27 NLT

I am leaving you with a gift—peace of mind and heart. And the peace I give is a gift the world cannot give. So don't be troubled or afraid.

The wise King Solomon states in Proverbs Chapter 3.

Proverbs 3:1-2 NLT

My child, never forget the things I have taught you.
Store my commands in your heart.
If you do this, you will live many years, and your life will be satisfying.

Now that I have told you about all these things that happen to your body when you have trouble dealing with the stress, fear, anger, worry, and anxiety of life, is there any evidence to support that having a God-centered paradigm makes a difference? If you are a Christian and have turned over your worry, fear, and anger over to God, are you healthier?

Let's take a look at the many medical studies about Christians living longer. There is more and more medical research at universities around the United States on the subject of religion and health. There is a tremendous amount of information and studies about whether Christians live longer. Dr. Bryon Johnson has reviewed over 770 studies on religion and health. His conclusion was that 85 percent of the studies show that faith in God has a beneficial effect. Dr. Johnson says that the studies show that if a person attends church on a regular basis, you can add seven years to your life if you are white—and fourteen years if you are black. Wow!

Go to www.webmd.com (which is the largest online medical website) and search "Go to Church, Live longer." You will find many studies and reports that show religion or God is associated with improved health and longer life spans.

Harold G. Koenig, M.D. of Duke University Medical Center in Durham, North Carolina has written several excellent books on Medicine, Health, and Religion. If you are interested in learning more about this subject, his books are a fabulous resource. He is the director of Duke University's Center for the Study of Religion, Spirituality, and Health. He has spent many years on the subjects of health, religion, and prayer.

In one of his studies it showed that people who attended religious services at least once a week were 46% less likely to die during the six years of the study. That is pretty remarkable! Another Duke University study of 2,391 people who were 65 years of age or older, who regularly attended church, who also prayed daily, or studied the Bible daily were 40% less likely to have high blood pressure than people who did not attend church. Dr. Koenig reviewed over 1,500 studies and concluded that people who are religious and pray more have better mental and physical health. He has also performed studies showing that prayer can have significant effect on hearing and vision improvement.

A study by David H. Rosmarin, PhD. at McLean Hospital and an instructor at Harvard Medical School showed that people with a strong or moderately strong belief in God had improved wellbeing, less depression, and were less likely to do self-harm. They also responded to treatment twice better that of non-believers. This is similar to the study I previously discussed about spiritual and Christian people have large brains, which was felt to give them better resistance to depression.

Tom Knox (a researcher and writer) was an atheist, but became a believer after doing in-depth research on the medical benefits of faith. Tom Knox states, "What I discovered astonished me. Over the past 30 years a growing and largely unnoticed body of scientific work shows religious belief is medically, socially, and psychologically beneficial."

San Francisco General Hospital looked at the effect of prayer on 393 cardiac patients. Half were prayed for by strangers who only had the patients' names. Those patients had fewer complications, fewer cases of pneumonia, and needed less medications.

As mentioned earlier, there are a large number of studies about Christians and health. The overwhelming majority of the studies show that being a Christian improves your health and that Christians live longer. The American Society of Hypertension stated that church-goers have lower blood pressure than non-believers.

The biggest step for many people is being able to turn everything over to God. For many people, they are unable to let go of all their negative emotions. You cannot let yourself lose control of all the aspects of your life. You have to be in charge. But, all the worries, fear, stress, and anger lead to an unhealthy level of anxiety. Like the hymn *I Surrender All,* you can decide to turn your life over to God and it will make a tremendous difference in your life. You will be happier, healthier, and have a close personal relationship with God's Holy Spirit. He is the ultimate doctor.

I will give you several Bible verses about how God wants us to live and later go over some health ideas that will help, as well.

Here are verses about **living life** every day.

Ecclesiastes 5:18-20 NLT

Even so, I have noticed one thing, at least, that is good. It is good for people to eat, drink, and enjoy their work under the sun during the short life God has given them, and to accept their lot in life. And it is a good thing to receive wealth from God and the good health to enjoy it. To enjoy your work and accept your lot in life- this is indeed a gift from God. God keeps such people busy enjoying life that they take no time to brood over the past.

These are Bible verses telling us not to **worry**. When I was growing up and upset or worried about something, my mother would always quote the Bible about not worrying. She said that God would take care of me and everything would turn out fine, according to God's plan. Anytime I start to worry about something happening in my life, I think about what she told me and the worry fades away.

Matthew 6:25-34 NLT

That is why I tell you not to worry about everyday life—whether you have enough food and drink, or enough clothes to wear. Isn't life more than food, and your body more than clothing? Look at the birds. They don't plant or harvest or store food in barns, for heavenly Father feeds them.

And aren't you far more valuable to him than they are? Can all your worries add a single moment to your life? And why worry about your clothing? Look at the lilies of the field and how they grow. They don't work or make their clothing, yet Solomon in all his glory was not dressed as beautiful as they are. And if God cares so wonderfully for wildflowers that are here today and thrown into the fire tomorrow, he will certainly care for you. Why do you have so little faith? So don't worry about these things, saying, What will we eat? What will we drink? What will we wear? These things dominate the thoughts of unbelievers, but your heavenly Father already knows your needs. Seek the Kingdom of God above all else, and live righteously, and he will give everything you need. So don't worry about tomorrow, for tomorrow will bring its own worries. Today's trouble is enough for today.

Philippians 4:6-7 NLT

Don't worry about anything; instead, pray about everything. Tell God what you need, and thank him for what he has done. Then you will experience God's peace, which exceeds anything that you can understand. His peace will guard your hearts and minds as you live in Christ Jesus.

Luke 12:25-26 NLT

Can all your worries add a single moment to your life? And if worry can't accomplish a little thing like that, what's the use of worrying over bigger things?

It is obvious that God does not want you to worry. You need to trust and have faith in Him to take care of you. He knows the damage worry does to your body and mind. Turn your worries over to Him.

The next verses are about **anger** and that you should control your anger and approach life differently.

James 1:20 NLT

Human anger does not produce the righteousness God desires.

Ephesians 4:26 NLT

And don't sin by letting anger control you. Don't let the sun go down while you are still angry,

Ephesians 4:31 NLT

Get rid of all bitterness, rage, anger, harsh words, and slander, as well as all types of evil behavior.

Proverbs 14:29 NLT

People with understanding control their anger; a hot temper shows great foolishness.

What does the Bible say about **fear**? Here are some Bible verses about fear.

Isaiah 41:10 NLV

Do not fear, for I am with you. Do not be afraid, for I am your God. I will give you strength, and for sure I will help you, Yes, I will hold you up with my right hand that is right and good.

2 Timothy 1:7 NLT

For God has not given us a spirit of fear and timidity, but of power, love, and self-discipline.

1 John 4:18 NLT

Such love has no fear, because perfect love expels all fear.

Hebrews 13:6 NLT

So we can say with confidence, The Lord is my helper, so I will have no fear.

Here are some other verses about **life and health**.

Proverbs 15:30 NLT

A cheerful look brings joy to the heart, good news makes for good health.

Isaiah 38:16 NLT

Lord your discipline is good, for it leads to life and health. You restore my health and allow me to live.

God is telling us to be disciplined in following His guidelines about health and mental attitude, which leads to life and health. The Bible is your guide or road map for your journey through life.

I have been giving you information about health, related to worry, stress, anger, and fear which leads to anxiety. This causes the release of free radicals in the body and oxidative stress. This causes damage to the cells of your body, including your brain.

Christians live longer than other people, as we discussed previously. I believe the reason for this is because many Christians have turned their life over to God. Christians handle the stress in life differently. They are calmer, as they have the peace and joy that God gives to His people. I believe Christians have less free radicals in their bodies. All the studies support or lead to this conclusion.

If you are struggling emotionally and need help with this, ask your pastor or see a Christian counselor.

What other things can you do to be healthy, once you have turned over your negative emotions to God? There many laws given by Moses in the Bible concerning health, sanitation, and how to live a healthy life. Let's take a look at what health and a diet from the Bible looks like.

What are the health laws of Moses and other health recommendations in the Bible? Are they scientifically based? Do they still apply today?

Moses's laws did not focus on treating disease, but focused on preventing disease and promoting health. Medical historian Ralph Major described Moses as the greatest sanitary engineer that the world has ever seen. Moses (or really God informing Moses) believed in the principle that prevention of disease is much simpler and invariably more far-reaching than the cure of disease.

Recent studies have indicated that our poor diets and lifestyle are responsible for up to 75% of cancers, heart disease, and stroke. There was one study that reported 90%. Approximately 50% of cancers are found in the organs of digestion. Paul Bragg in his famous cookbook said, "The average person is poisoning himself day by day with the food he eats." Nearly 50 % of Americans are obese or overweight. Nearly thirty million people in the United States have diabetes. The rate at which people are newly diagnosed with diabetes has tripled in the last thirty years.

Does God care if you are healthy, happy, and live a long life?
3 John 1:2 NLT

Dear friend, I pray that you are in good health and that all may go well with you even as your soul is getting along well.

Exodus 23:25 NLT

You must serve only the Lord your God. If you do, I will bless you with food and water, and I will protect you from illness.

1 Corinthians 10:31 NLT

So whether you eat or drink, or whatever you do, do it all for the glory of God.

1 Corinthians 6:19-20 NLT

Don't you realize that your body is the temple of the Holy Spirit, who lives in you and was given to you by God? You do not belong to yourself, for God bought you with a high price. So you must honor God with your body.

It appears that God cares about your health and well-being. He gave us all kinds of advice about health in the Bible. I am not going to cover all the laws in the Bible, but let's explore some of God's health advice.

First, look at our teeth structure. Our teeth were not designed by God to eat meat. If someone has just killed a big water buffalo, are you able to go there and bite a big hunk of shoulder off of it? No, our teeth are not like that of a carnivore with sharp pointed teeth to tear meat. Our teeth look more like animals that are vegetarians, such as a cow or lamb. In the Garden of Eden, Adam and Eve ate from seed-bearing plants.

Genesis 1:29 NLT

Then God said, Look! I have given you every seed-bearing plant throughout the earth and all the fruit trees for your food.

After sinning and being forced out of the Garden of Eden, God gave Adam and Eve new instructions for living their lives.

Health Benefits of a God-Centered Paradigm

Genesis 3:17-19 NLT

Cursed is the ground because of you; through painful toil you will eat food from it all the days of your life. It will produce thorns and thistles for you, and you will eat the plants of the field. By the sweat of your brow you will eat your food.

Adam and Eve, along with the other people of the world, were vegetarians.

With the great flood God gave Noah new instructions about eating.

Genesis 7:2 NLT

Take with you 7 pairs-male and female- of each animal I have approved for eating and for sacrifice, and take 1 pair of each of the others.

God told Noah that he could eat meat. Noah was on the ark for nearly one year.

There would not be any way to keep vegetables fresh on the ark for that long without refrigeration. There would be no crops after the flood and they would have to cultivate new crops. God did limit the types of meat that they could eat. God knew that certain animals could contain a variety of diseases and could be contaminated.

People lived to be very old in the beginning. Adam lived to 920, Enoch to 905, and Noah lived 950 years. God was not happy with the way man lived and decided to limit the number of years we live to 120. We still have the potential to live that long; but very rarely does someone live anywhere near that long today. The question is whether our life style and diet is limiting our life span? I believe that there is good evidence that it is. There is a tremendous amount of evidence to support it.

Adam and Eve would have never developed cancer, diabetes, high blood pressure, heart attacks or strokes in my opinion. Ever since they sinned and were thrown out of Eden, man has turned away from God's teachings. All the thousands of years of not following God's health directives has led us to the health condition we find ourselves in today. There are studies that show that lifestyle is responsible for up to 75% of deaths. People who smoke, are overweight, or consume too much alcohol are causing their own demise. I have seen one study that states the number is 90%. God did not create cancer, we did. God wanted his people to be healthy and be an example to other people in the world. The people of God would live longer and stay healthier.

God gave Moses laws that His people should live by. These laws were for their health. The people of that time did not know the scientific or medical reasons for the laws. They just knew that God told them to follow them.

Look at our health today in America. The average diet that Americans eat today is horrible. We are bombarded with advertising about this food or this restaurant. We have eating contests to see who can eat the most food. A shocking 25 percent of adults over age 65 have diabetes. The incidence of diabetes is rising rapidly in the United States, because of our diets and lifestyle. Moses' diet laws are found in Leviticus 11 and Deuteronomy 14.

You may eat any land animal that has completely split hooves and chews the cud. You may eat ox, sheep, goat, deer, gazelle, roe deer, wild goat, addax, antelope, and mountain sheep. You may not eat the camel, hyrax, hare, and pig. The animals that we are not to eat are because they have a higher incidence of carrying diseases.

Of the marine animals, you may eat anything from the water that has both fins and scales. You may not eat catfish, eels, lobsters, clams, oysters, shrimp, frogs, and others. The marine animals that you are not to eat tend to be bottom feeders, filter feeders, and are more likely to carry disease.

Health Benefits of a God-Centered Paradigm

These birds are not to be eaten. The griffon vulture, bearded vulture, black vulture, kite, falcons of all kinds, ravens of all kinds, eagle owl, short-eared owl, seagull, hawks of all kinds, owls, herons, and bats. Again, these birds tend to carry disease.

You must not eat insects that walk on the ground. You may eat winged insects that walk on the ground and have jointed legs so they can jump. They are locusts, bald locusts, crickets, and grasshoppers. You can have all these roasted that you care to eat! Small animal that scurry along the ground you may not eat. The mole rat, rat, large lizards of all kinds, gecko, monitor lizard, common lizard, sand lizard, and chameleon. These animals also carry diseases.

You may ask, Do these health laws still need to be followed? In the last chapter of Isaiah 66 which is about the second coming of Christ, verse 17 gives a warning. *Those who 'consecrate' and 'purify' themselves in a sacred garden with its idol in the center—feasting on pork and rats, and other detestable meats—will come to a terrible end,"* says the Lord.

Maybe these health laws need to be followed still today! If you look at the sanitary and health conditions in third world countries, it is deplorable. If they just followed the laws of Moses, their living conditions and health could be miraculously changed.

We have our own issues with the food in the United States. Cattle are given 29 million pounds of antibiotics a year. Seventy percent of the antibiotics in the United States is given to animals. Fifty percent of antibiotics given to humans is unnecessary and taken incorrectly. Most colds are caused by a virus and antibiotics are not effective against a virus. Also, we stop the antibiotics as soon as we are feeling better which gives the bacteria a chance to develop resistance to the antibiotic as we did not completely kill all the bacteria. The bacteria are being exposed to antibiotics too much and not in a proper manner. Antibiotic resistant bacteria are becoming much more prevalent due to this practice. MCR-1 is a gene mutation that allows the bacteria to become resistant to nearly all antibiotics. It is spreading rapidly from bacteria to bacteria. In the grocery store, 81 percent of ground turkey, 66 percent of pork chops, 55 percent of ground beef, and 39 percent of chicken contain antibiotic resistant bacteria. As you see, our food today has its problems.

Some of the other health laws in the Bible are:

You must not eat anything that has died a natural cause. You don't know what it died from.

You must never eat fat or blood.

All human waste had to be disposed of outside of the home and city.

There were laws concerning quarantine for people with illnesses and laws about touching someone who had died.

There were laws about the warriors not coming back home immediately after battle. They could bring some disease home to their families. They had to remain away and clean all their metal battle gear and any metal bounty through fire. They had to wash their clothes, and other perishable materials in water twice in the seven days, while they were to remain away from home. All these health laws were made for the people of Israel to follow as a protection for them. The people of Israel were healthier and stronger than their neighbors. They had no knowledge of bacteria or viruses and just followed God's laws.

Antony van Leeuwenhoek is the father of microbiology and discovered bacteria in 1676. Louis Pasteur didn't propose the relationship of bacteria to disease until the 1860s. Alexander Fleming and Edward Jenner were the first to prove the existence of viruses, with the invention of the electron microscope in 1930. The laws that God gave to Moses were based on science. He knew about the bacteria and viruses that He created. God told Moses which foods and animals that were safe to eat. The question is, do they still apply today?

As I related before, if you are living in a third world country, these laws would improve the health of the people living there. It is a shame that they don't follow His laws. God wants His people to be healthy. There are thousands of studies about this diet or that diet. Man devised diets are just their opinion or a way to make money by writing a book. Diets never work. Living a lifestyle does work. There are some well accepted health recommendations that you should follow.

There is a book by Dan Buettner called *The Blue Zones Solution: The Revolutionary Plan to Eat and Live your Way Lifelong Health*. It is about the areas of the world where the highest percentage of people live to over 100 years of age. These areas of the world are called *blue zones*. From his research, the author believes that anyone can add 12 years to their life by following the principles common to the people living in these zones.

There is another book that I read several years ago before the Blue Zone book was published called *The Okinawa Program* by Bradley and Craig Willcox and Makoto Suzuki. This book is about a 25-year study of the people of Okinawa. Okinawa is one of the blue zones. The book gives details of their lifestyles, culture, and diet which enables them to live long healthy lives.

The blue zones of the world are Ikaria, Greece; Sardinia, Italy; Nicoya Peninsula, Costa Rica; Okinawa, Japan; and Loma Linda, California. There are some common things between all the different areas of the world that benefit one's health. The words in parenthesis are mine.

- Have goals in life
- Decrease stress (as discussed previously)
- Eat less (Americans especially eat too much)
- Limited amounts of meat
- Have faith (Christians live longer)

- Stay social (Have close Christian friends)
- Love for spouse and family
- Exercise, but at more moderate levels—which could be walking or working in the yard daily.
- Glass of red wine a day (This may be against some beliefs, such as the Seventh-Day Adventists in Loma Linda; but wine was a factor in the other blue zones. Also, there is concern that some people may not be able to limit their wine consumption.)
- The people of Okinawa drink miso soup like we drink coffee. They also eat a lot of a Japanese sweet potato. The people in Greece and Sardinia follow the Mediterranean diet which is vegetables, legumes (beans, peas, and lentils), fruits, cereals or grains, fish, nuts, and mono-unsaturated fats (olive oil).

Another great book about diet and health is the *Super Immunity: The Essential Nutrition Guide for Boosting Your Body's Defenses to Live Longer* by Joel Fuhrman, M.D. This book gives a lot of scientific medical information about eating healthy and how it affects the body and its immune system.

He recommends a vegetarian diet composed of cruciferous vegetable, nuts, seeds, beans, fruits, and legumes. Cruciferous vegetables received their name for their flowers which have four equally spaced petals in the shape of a cross. Hence the Latin word *crucifer* which means cross-bearer. It is interesting that the healthiest plants that you can eat have a flower shaped like a cross. God is amazing in the finite details in which He has made this world that we live in. Cruciferous vegetables are kale, cabbage, collards, broccoli, cauliflower, and turnips.

If you are going to eat animal protein, then Dr. Fuhrman says to limit it to 3 or 4 ounces a day. There is a hormone called IGF-1 or insulin-like growth factor. It is necessary in your body. It is especially important for growth and development as you grow. If you are an athlete, it is important to build muscle mass and strength. After reaching adulthood, there are studies that show high levels in the body are harmful. Adults with lower levels live longer. Eating large amounts of animal protein will raise the level of IGF-1 in the body. A high level of this hormone in the body means a shorter life span. Lower levels result in a longer life span. This is consistent with the diets of people who live in the blue zones. They all eat small portions of protein and usually it is fish.

If what I have been saying is true about health and God, then where is having a God-centered paradigm concerning a blue zone. Guess what, one of the blue zones is a religion. One of the blue zones is Loma Linda, California and the home of many Seventh-Day Adventists. There have been numerous scientific studies on their life-styles, faith, and health. You don't need to be a member of the Seventh-Day Adventists to learn from them about living longer and healthier lives.

One of the main beliefs of Seventh-Day Adventists is that your body is not your own. This point of view comes from the Bible. Remember the Bible verses about your body is the temple of God. Another Bible verse about this is.

1 Corinthians 3:16-17 NLT

Don't you realize that all of you together are the temple of God and that the Spirit of God lives in you? God will destroy anyone who destroys this temple. For God's temple is holy, and you are that temple.

You can see from these Bible verses that your body is a temple where the Holy Spirit resides in you. If your lifestyle is not according to God's desires, you are defiling His temple. The Seventh-Day Adventist follow these Scriptures of the Bible. The McDonalds in Loma Linda has as its main item on their menu a veggie burger. A popular item in the grocery stores is Tofu Links or Tofu hot dogs. Sugar is taboo, as well. The cafeteria at Loma Linda University is vegetarian.

Death rates from cancer among Seventh-Day Adventists is 60% lower for men and 76% lower for women. Coronary artery disease is lower, especially for men with as much as a 60% decrease. There is approximately a 70% decrease in respiratory disease.

Their diets are vegetarian in that they eat fruits, vegetables, legumes, whole grains, nuts, dairy products, and olive oil. They do not smoke, use alcohol, and keep away from caffeine.

In Nicoya Peninsula, Costa Rica a large portion of their diet is composed of beans, squash, and corn. Plus, they eat yams and fruits such as bananas, papayas, and peach palms.

In the United States today, we don't have to be as concerned about food being contaminated as in the Old Testament, because our food is inspected. There are outbreaks of contamination on some occasions, but not very often.

Having a God-centered paradigm means living longer and having better health. There are approximately 2,000 studies that show Christians live six to seven years longer than non-Christians. Like the MasterCard commercials about value, God's healthcare plan is priceless. God wants you to be healthy. What you put into your body does make a difference.

Proverbs 17:22 NLT

A cheerful heart is good medicine. Living a life where our worries and fears are turned over to God gives us peace and joy.

Ecclesiastes 3:13 NLT

And people should eat and drink and enjoy the fruits of their labor, for these are gifts from God.

Another important factor in living a long healthy life is **moderation or discipline**.

Philippians 4:5 KJV

Let your moderation be known unto all men.

Health Benefits of a God-Centered Paradigm

1 Corinthians 9:25 NLT

All athletes are disciplined in their training. They do it to win a prize that will fade away, but we do it for an eternal prize.

God's Health Plan

Forget about all these diets that are promoted by this person or that person. The vast amount of documentation about the health benefits of a Mediterranean style diet is undeniable. It agrees with the recommendations in the Bible.

You need to do things in life with moderation and use discipline to keep you focused on your journey through life. The best thing you can do is turn over your life to God. He has a plan specially planned for you.

Release your worries, fear, stress, anger, and anxiety to the ultimate healer God. These negative emotions are the great killer in the United States. God wants you to hand them over to Him.

Begin to eat a good diet, like the Mediterranean diet with vegetables, fruits, beans, olive oil, legumes, nuts, lentils, and a reduced amount of animal protein in the area of 3 to 4 ounces per day. One of your meals should be a large green salad with fruit, seeds, and nuts. I usually eat this for lunch.

Limit your portion sizes of food. You can eat as much salad as you want, but just be careful with the dressing.

Moderate exercise four times a week. You don't have to be a fitness fanatic.

Follow the other recommendations from the people who live in the blue zones.

God gave us the first recipe for a health food bar or bread in the Bible.

Ezekiel 4:9 NLT

Now go and get some wheat, barley, beans, lentils, millet, and emmer wheat, and mix them together in a storage jar. Use them to make bread for yourself.

Living life with a God-centered paradigm means taking care of your body with turning over your life to God; releasing your worries, fears, anger, stress, and anxiety to Him; and eating a healthy diet and moderate exercise. This is not rocket science. It is doable by everyone. God is ready to help. The great news is that you will be healthier. You will live six to seven years longer or maybe more. God's health plan is the only one you should follow.

John 15:11 NLT

I have told you these things so that you will be filled with my joy. Yes, your joy will overflow.

Psalms 67:2 NLT

May your ways be known throughout the earth. You saving power among people everywhere.

John 10:10

My purpose is to give them a rich and satisfying life.

Your health and life should be centered around God's plan for you. He has an awesome plan for each of you.

Sign up for God's healthcare plan!

Chapter 6
Spiritual Benefits of a God-Centered Paradigm

Galatians 5:22 NLT

But the Holy Spirit produces this kind of fruit in our lives: love, joy, peace, patience, kindness, goodness, faithfulness, gentleness, and self-control.

I have written this chapter is a different manner. I am going to cover each of the fruits of the Spirit beginning with a common definition. This will be followed by the Greek word for each fruit, as sometimes the Greek word gives a more complete meaning or fuller explanation. I am going to follow that with synonyms for each fruit, as this can help deepen and broaden the meaning of the word. There will be Bible verses that correspond to each fruit of the spirit. Then some of my own insights will be added to the text. One of the major benefits of a God-centered paradigm is that the fruit of the Spirit will become a dominant feature of your soul or personality. The fruit of the Spirit will change you spiritually and physically (health).

When you have accepted Jesus Christ as your Lord and Savior, you receive the Holy Spirit. The Holy Spirit takes up living quarters inside you.

2 Corinthians 5:17 NLT

This means that anyone who belongs to Christ has become a new person. The old life is gone; a new life has begun!

In others words, you have a new paradigm—a God-centered paradigm. The Holy Spirit then will start to produce in you a new way of living your life. The Holy Spirit gives you two things that affect your life: the gifts of the Holy Spirit and the fruit of the Holy Spirit. The gifts are abilities and manifestations empowered to us. The gifts are speaking in tongues, interpretation of tongues, prophecy, knowledge, words of wisdom, discerning of spirits, faith, healing, and miracles. I am not going to go into detail about the gifts, as they are the given abilities by the Holy Spirit.

The fruit of the Spirit is about how you will live your life. You become a new creature or person. You have a new paradigm to live your life by.

Matthew 7:16-20 NLT

Beware of false prophets who come disguised as harmless sheep but are really vicious wolves. You can identify them by their fruit, that is, by the way they act. Can you pick grapes from thorn bushes, or figs from thistles? A good tree produces good fruit, and a bad tree produces bad fruit. So every tree that does not produce good fruit is chopped down and thrown into the fire. Yes, just as you can identify a tree by its fruit, so you can identify people by their actions.

The fruit of the Holy Spirit will be center stage now. As I have discussed before, your mind tends to work in a way to satisfy your personal and selfish needs. You can find yourself stuck in a quagmire of negative thoughts and emotions. Many people keep stimulating their amygdala and limbic system, which is bad for their health and mental well-being. This prevents you from using your prefrontal cortex properly. Therefore, people make bad decisions throughout much of their lives.

John Chapter 14 tells us that all who love Him will do what He says. Then the Father will love us and we come to each of them. God sends His Holy Spirit as His representative and advocate. The Holy Spirit will teach you everything and remind you of everything.

Spiritual Benefits of a God-Centered Paradigm

Let's see what it says in the Bible about living your life guided by the Holy Spirit.

Galatians 5:16-26 NLT

So I say, let the Holy Spirit guide your lives. Then you won't be doing what your sinful nature craves. The sinful nature wants to do evil, which is just the opposite of what the Spirit wants. And the Spirit gives us desires that are opposite of what the sinful nature desires. These two forces are constantly fighting each other, so you are not free to carry out your good intentions. But when you are directed by the Spirit, you are not under obligation to the law of Moses. When you follow the desires of your sinful nature, the results are very clear; sexual immorality, impurity, lustful pleasures, idolatry, sorcery, hostility, quarreling, jealously, outbursts of anger, selfish ambition, dissention, division, envy, drunkenness, wild parties, and other sins like these. (my insertion; you keep stimulating your amygdala and limbic system which leads to these and other things such as worry, depression, stress, anxiety, and fear) *Let me tell you again, as I have before, that anyone living that sort of life will not inherit the Kingdom of God. But the Holy Spirit produces this kind of fruit in our lives: love, joy, peace, patience, kindness, goodness, faithfulness, gentleness, and self-control. There is no law against these things!*

Those who belong to Christ Jesus have nailed the passions and desires of their sinful nature to his cross and crucified them there. Since we are living by the Spirit, let us follow the Spirit's leading in every part of our lives. Let us not become conceited, or provoke another, or be jealous of one another.

John 14:25-26 NLT

I am telling you these things now while I am still with you. But when the Father sends the Advocate as my representative—that is, the Holy Spirit—he will teach you everything and will remind you of everything I have told you.

Let's go through the different fruit of the Spirit and see what having them means to your life.

Joy

Joy as defined by Merriam-Webster is:
- *A feeling of great happiness;*
- *A source or cause of delight;*
- *Success in doing, finding, or getting something;*
- *The emotion evoked by well-being, success, or good fortune or by the prospect of processing what one desires.*

The Greek word for joy is *Chara*. This means cheerfulness or calm delight or gladness. Chara is the joy and happiness experienced as a result of grace which brings well-being.

Synonyms for joy: happy, glad, cheerful, rejoicing, delight, satisfaction, pleasure, glee, exuberance, elation, bliss

Joy is a state or condition in your mind and heart (soul). There are many ways to define it, such as from a dictionary. But the joy from the Holy Spirit is not just an emotion, a laugh, a smile, or fleeting thought, it is something more substantial or deeper. It is something that is permanent. The joy of the Holy Spirit is not temporary. A portion of it is knowing that God wants you to be joyful. Knowing that you are going to spend eternity in Heaven with God is beyond fantastic or amazing. You should always be joyful since your final destination is Heaven.

Rick Warren's definition of joy is *the settled assurance that God is in control of all details of my life, the quiet confidence that ultimately everything is going to be alright, and the determined choice to praise God in every situation.*

Acts 13:52 NLT

And the believers were filled with joy and with the Holy Spirit.

Romans 4:7 NLT

Oh, what joy for those whose disobedience is forgiven, whose sins are put out of sight.

Romans 14:17 NLT

For the Kingdom of God is not a matter of what we eat or drink, but of living a life of goodness and peace and joy in the Holy Spirit.

Romans 5:2 NLT

Because of our faith, Christ has brought us into this place of undeserved privilege where we now stand, and we confidently and joyfully look forward to sharing God's glory.

1 John 1:4 KJV

And those things we write to you that your joy may be full.

Read the Bible every day and be full of joy every day!!!

Peace

Peace as defined by Merriam-Webster:
- A state of tranquility or quiet;
- Freedom from civil disturbance;
- Freedom from disquieting or oppressive thoughts or emotions;
- Harmony in personal relations;

The Greek word for peace is *Eirene* and the Hebrew word is *Shalom*. Eirene means the rule of order in place of chaos. The idea of wholeness or tranquility that is not affected by the outside world. Shalom is more than just peace. It is a complete peace, harmony, contentment, well-being, perfect, complete, and full.

Synonyms for peace: freedom from war, harmony, concord, serenity, tranquility, calm, undisturbed state of mind, absence of anxiety, absence of mental conflict, contentment.

Having peace in your mind can diminish the stimulation of your limbic system and quiet your brain and body. Your prefrontal cortex will function more efficiently. This is the first step for people who are struggling with mental issues. The peace of God calming your mind is essential. God wants you to be at peace both internally and externally.

Acts 10:36 NLT

This is the message of Good News for the people of Israel—that there is peace with God through Jesus Christ, who is Lord of all.

John 16:33 NLT

I have told you all this so that you may have peace in me. Here on earth you will have many trials and sorrows. But take heart, because I have overcome the world.

John 14:27

I am leaving you with a gift—peace of mind and heart. And the peace I give is a gift the world cannot give. So don't be troubled or afraid.

Many people think that they are in charge of everything in their lives. From the verses above, you can see that God is actually in charge. For the people dealing with depression, anxiety, and the other negative emotions, this is one of the keys to changing their lives.

Accept the peace of the Holy Spirit and release your stress, fear, worry, and anxiety!

Patience

Patient or patience as defined by Merriam-Webster:

- Able to remain calm and not become annoyed when waiting for a long period of time or when dealing with problems or difficult people.
- Done in a careful way over a long period of time without hurrying.

The Greek word for patience is actually two words *makrothumia* and *hupomone*. Makrothumia comes from *makros* meaning long and *thumos* meaning temper. The word means forbearance, patient endurance, and long suffering. Hupomone means endurance. Hupomone comes from *hupo* under and *mone* to remain. It means to withstand difficult circumstances.

Synonyms for patience: tolerance, endurance, resolve, forbearance, restraint, self-restraint, composure, stoicism, understanding, perseverance

We live in a world where everyone wants instant gratification and rewards.

Technology and the internet allows immediate contact and exposure to unlimited things, resources, and information. The person with the most toys wins.

As I have discussed many times before, all this stimulation is not good for your mind and body. You worry and become anxious because something does not meet your time schedule. You need to slow down your life and spend quiet time. God rested on the seventh day and you are supposed to rest on the seventh day. Demanding instant rewards and gratification is not what the Bible teaches.

James 1:2-8 NLT

Dear brothers and sisters, when troubles of any kind come your way, consider it an opportunity for great joy. For you know when your faith is tested, your endurance has a chance to grow. So let it grow, for when your endurance is fully developed, you will be perfect and complete, needing

nothing. If you need wisdom, ask our generous God, and he will give it to you. He will not rebuke you for asking. But when you ask him, be sure that your faith is in God alone. Do not waver, for person with divided loyalty is as unsettled as a wave of the sea that is blown and tossed by the wind. Such people should not expect to receive anything from the Lord. Their loyalty is divided between God and the world, and they are unstable in everything they do.

James 1:12 NLT

God blesses those who patiently endure testing and temptation.

Colossians 3:12 NLT

Since God chose you to be the holy people he loves, you must clothe yourselves with tenderhearted mercy, kindness, gentleness, and patience.

Ecclesiastes 7:8 NLT

Finishing is better than starting. Patience is better than pride.

2 Corinthians 6:6 NLT

We prove ourselves by our purity, our understanding, our patience, our kindness, by the Holy Spirit within us, and by our sincere love.

As in the old saying, good things come to those who wait, put yourself on God's time!

Kindness

Kindness as defined by Merriam-Webster:

- A kind deed;
- A kind act;
- The quality or state of being kind;

The Greek word for kindness is *chrestotes*. Chrestotes means to show kindness or friendliness to others.

Synonyms for chrestotes: sympathy, compassion, benevolence, tenderheartedness, generosity, mercy, charity

Having a kind disposition changes how you treat others, but also calms you down as well. Jesus' new commandment is that you are to love your neighbors as you love yourself. That means you need to be kind to others. It shows other people that the Holy Spirit is involved in your life. If everyone was kind in this world, it would be a much different place. God thinks that being kind is an important part of living the way He wants you to live.

2 Corinthians 6:1 NLT

As God's partners, we beg you not to accept this marvelous gift of God's kindness and then ignore it.

2 Corinthians 6:6 NLT

We prove ourselves by our purity, our understanding, our patience, our kindness, by the Holy Spirit within us, and by our sincere love.

Philippians 4:17 NLT

I don't say this because I want a gift from you. Rather, I want you to receive a reward for your kindness.

Romans 12:8 NLT

If your gift is to encourage others, be encouraging. If it is giving, give generously. If God has given you leadership ability, take the responsibility seriously. And if you have a gift for showing kindness to others, do it gladly.

My mother used to tell me an old country saying. "Son, you get more flies with honey than with vinegar." Develop a kind attitude that will please God. People will see that you are different, you are a Christian. You are witness for God, just by showing kindness to others. Being kind will benefit you personally as well, as it will help calm your mind. It is hard to be amped up while showing kindness.

Be kind, it feels great!

Goodness

Goodness as defined by Merriam-Webster:

- The quality or state of being good;

The Greek word for goodness is *agathosune*. Agathosune means uprightness of heart and life. Another meaning of goodness from the word agathosune is zealous activity in doing good.

Synonyms for goodness: virtue, righteousness, morality, purity, warmth, nobility, respectability, decency, honor, truth, truthfulness

The word good is used in a wide variety of situations and contexts. We use it so frequently and nonchalantly that it can lose its true meaning, especially Biblically. I might think that something tastes good and another person may think that it tastes fair, poor, or badly. Good should have some implication of some degree of excellence. Goodness suggests a quality that is desirable, something commendable, beneficial, enjoyable, exemplary, or admirable. It should not be a passive process, but an active process. You are to be actively or zealously pursuing goodness especially to others.

1 Peter 2:9 NLT

But you are not like that, for you are a chosen people.
You are royal priests, a holy nation, God's very own possession.
As a result, you can show others the goodness of God,
for He called you out of the darkness into His wonderful light.

Romans 8:28 NLT

And we know that God causes everything to work together for the good of those who love God and are called according to his purpose for them.

Romans 14:17 NLT

For the Kingdom of God is not a matter of what we eat or drink, but of living a life of goodness and peace and joy.

We are to show others goodness, as God has been good to us. By our example of being good and treating others with love, we are shining God's light into a dark world.

Be good for goodness sake!

Faithfulness

Faithfulness as defined by Merriam-Webster:
- Having or showing true and constant support or loyalty;
- Deserving trust; keeping your promises or doing what you are supposed to do;
- Steadfast in affection or allegiance;
- Firm in adherence to promises or in observance of duty.

The Greek word for faithfulness is *pistis*. Pistis means to persuade or be persuaded, which is the core meaning of faith as being" divine persuasion" received from God. It is also the characteristic of the man who is reliable. In Hebrew faithful is *emunah,* which means firmness or fidelity.

Synonyms for faithfulness: passionate, serious, ardent, resolute, unwavering, responsible, dedicated, devoted, devout, good, loyal, staunch, steadfast, true, dependable, dutiful, reliable

Your normal human characteristics are centered around you and what you want. What pleasures or things do you want for yourself? In that context, how can a person be faithful to God when many people love themselves more? Through the help of the Holy Spirit, you have to decide on what you value or is truly important and then commit yourself to it.

2 Timothy 2:22 NLT

Run from anything that stimulate youthful lusts. Instead,

pursue righteous living, faithfulness, love, and peace. Enjoy the companionship of those who call on the Lord with pure hearts.

1 Timothy 1:19 NLT

Cling to your faith in Christ, and keep your conscience clear.

Psalm 92:2 NLT

It is good to proclaim your unfailing love in the morning, your faithfulness in the evening.

Luke 16:10 NLT

If you are faithful in little things, you will be faithful in large ones.

Luke 17:6 NLT

The Lord answered, "If you had the faith even as small as a mustard seed, you could say to this mulberry tree, 'May you be uprooted and thrown into the sea, and it would obey you!"

If you have faith in that Jesus Christ is your Lord and Savior, then through the strength of the Holy Spirit work at being faithful every day.

Hebrews 11:1-3 MSG

The fundamental fact of existence is that this trust in God, this faith, is the firm foundation under everything that makes life worth living. It's our handle on what we can't see. The act of faith is what distinguished our ancestors, set them above the crowd. By Faith, we see the world called into existence by God's word, what we see created by what we don't see.

O come all ye faithful joyful and triumphant

O come ye. O come ye to Bethlehem

Come and behold him!

Gentleness

Gentleness as defined by Merriam-Webster:

- Having or showing a kind and quiet nature: not harsh or violent;
- Not hard or forceful;
- Not strong or harsh in effect or quality.

The Greek word for gentleness is *prautes*. Prautes means mildness, gentleness, or meekness. It is having a disposition of gentleness.

Synonyms for gentleness: good-natured, humane, lenient, merciful, mild, tender, sympathetic, considerate, understanding, compassionate, benevolent, serene, sweet-tempered.

When you first think about the word gentleness, you think about someone being weak. In today's world where rap music describes horrible things such as killing and rape, does anyone think that gentleness still applies in today's society? People are all about winning and doing whatever it takes to win. It is all about me and you don't think about others.

Christians should treat other people differently than non-Christians. Gentleness means treating others with kindness, tenderness, understanding, and putting yourself aside to help others in need. God was not happy with the proud, like the Pharisees in the Bible, but gives grace to the humble and kind.

Philippians 4:5 NLT

Let everyone see that you are considerate in all you do.

1 Corinthians 4:20-21 NLT

For the Kingdom of God is not just talk; it is living by God's power. Which do you choose? Should I come with a rod to punish you, or should I come with love and a gentle spirit?

2 Timothy 2:24-25 NLT

A servant of the Lord must not quarrel but must be kind to everyone, be able to teach, and be patient with difficult people. Gently instruct those who oppose truth. Perhaps God will change those people's hearts, and they will learn the truth.

1 Peter 3:15-16 NLT

Instead, you must worship Christ as Lord of your life. And if someone asks about your hope as a believer, always be ready to explain it. But do this in a gentle and respectful way.

As I stated above, gentleness is considered weak and something that many people would choose not to embrace. Having a gentle spirit from the Holy Spirit requires strength, determination, and self-control, in order to be effective as a witness to others. It takes a strong person to show gentleness to others. Jesus lived a life of gentleness even though He had the power to do anything He wanted.

Saint Frances de Sales has a quote about gentleness.

*Nothing is so strong as gentleness,
nothing so gentle as real strength.*

Be gentle!

Self-Control

Self-Control as defined by Merriam-Webster:

- Restraint exercised over one's own impulses, emotions, or desires;
- The ability to control oneself especially in tough or difficult circumstances;

The Greek word for self-control is *egkrareia*. Power over oneself, self-mastery, able to control one's thoughts.

Spiritual Benefits of a God-Centered Paradigm

Synonyms for self-control: restraint, moderation, self-discipline, self-command, self-possession, will power, composure, temperance

Self-control obviously can be very difficult to actually do. More than fifty percent of Americans are overweight, which is the result of poor self-control. All the crime in America in many ways is related to poor self-control. Developing self-control is not only advantageous for us personally, but it affects how we treat others as well.

The ultimate example of self-control was Jesus. He came to earth and took on the form of man. He faced all the same temptations we do and more. He spent forty days in the desert being tempted by the devil. He had perfect self-control.

Proverbs 5:23 NLT

He will die for lack of self-control; he will be lost because of his great foolishness.

Proverbs 25:28 NLT

A person without self-control is like a city with broken-down walls.

1 Peter 1:13 NLT

So prepare your minds for action and exercise self-control.

2 Peter 5:7 NLT

In view of all this, make every effort to respond to God's promises.

Supplement your faith with a generous provision of moral excellence, and moral excellence with knowledge, and knowledge with self-control, and self-control with patient endurance, and patient endurance with godliness, and godliness with brotherly affection, and brotherly affection with love for everyone.

Self-control is a constant battle in our lives and the Holy Spirit is our strength. A quote by Lane Olinghouse is: *Those who flee temptation, generally leave a forwarding address.*

Have self-control front and center in your life!

Love

I decided to discuss the spiritual fruit of love last, even though it was listed first in Galatians 5:22. I believe it is the most important fruit of the Spirit. Paul writes in Colossians, *That above all, clothe yourselves with love, which binds us all together in perfect harmony.*

Love as defined by Merriam-Webster:

- A feeling of strong or constant affection for a person;
- Attraction that includes sexual desire: the strong affection felt by people who have a romantic relationship;
- A person you love in a romantic way;

The Greek word for love that describes the kind of love God has for you and wants you to have, is *agape*. Agape is the highest form of love, which is a selfless, undefeatable, never wavering, benevolence, and committed passionately towards the well-being of others. Another term would be charity.

Synonyms for love: Fondness, tenderness, worship, attachment, passion, infatuation, romance, goodwill, compassion, warmth, devotion, ardor, caring, sympathy, intimacy, adoration, lust, friendliness, doting, yearning.

As with the word good, the word love is used very loosely in today's society. We love chocolate, football, TV, movies, sleep, movie stars, and food. The list could go on forever. Today people think that love is this warm fuzzy feeling, a tightness in the chest, a twinge in the stomach, or a tingly feeling that runs up and down the spine.

The fruit of the spirit related to love is a specific type of love which is called agape in the Bible. There are four Greek words for love found in the Bible which are *eros, storge, philos,* and *agape*. The word love appears in the NLT Bible 759 times. God must think it is pretty important.

Philos is the kind of love you have for a friend or companion. It is loving someone like a brother or sister. This is the love for a close friend.

But this type of love can be temporary or change. You have close friend in high school that later in life you no longer have a relationship with them.

Eros is the Greek word referring to desire, longing, or lust. It refers to erotic love. Eros is the Greek god of love. Obviously this type of love can be very fleeting, as some people are in this type of love and suddenly they don't love that person anymore.

Storge is the Greek word for family love. It is the love between mothers, fathers, sons, daughters, brothers, and sisters. It is cherishing one's kindred, love based on one's own nature, or loving affection. It is the quiet feeling of having a loved one close to you.

Agape, as I defined in the beginning, is a different type of love. Agape is a selfless, dependable, constant, and self-sacrificing love or caring for someone. It is dependable, constant, never wavering, not based on emotions. It is a mental commitment made to someone permanently. This the type of love you are to have for God and other people.

Matthew 22:39-39 NLT

Jesus replied, 'You must love the Lord your God with all your heart, all your soul, and all your mind.' This is the first and greatest commandment. A second is equally important: 'Love your neighbor as yourself.'

John 14:23 NLT

Jesus replied, 'All who love me will do what I say. My Father will love them, and we will come and make our home with each of them.'

Romans 12:9-10 NLT

Don't just pretend to love others. Really love them. Hate what is wrong. Hold tightly to what is good. Love each other with genuine affection, and take delight in honoring each other.

Colossians 3:12-14 NLT

Since God chose you to be the holy people he loves, you must clothe yourselves with tenderhearted mercy, kindness, humility, gentleness, and patience. Make allowance for each other's faults, and forgive anyone who offends you. Remember, the Lord forgave you, so you must forgive others. Above all, clothe yourselves with love, which binds us all together in perfect harmony.

1 Corinthians 13:1-13 NLT

If I could speak all the languages of earth and of angels, but didn't love others, I would only be a noisy gong or clanging cymbal. If I had the gift of prophecy, and if I understood all of God's secret plans and possessed all knowledge, and if I had such faith that I could move mountains, but didn't love others, I would be nothing. If I gave everything I have to the poor and even sacrificed my body, I could boast about it; but if I didn't love others, I would have gained nothing.

Love is patient and kind. Love is not jealous or boastful or proud or rude. It does not demand its own way. It is not irritable, and it keeps no record of being wronged. It does not rejoice about injustice but rejoices whenever the truth wins out. Love never gives up, never loses faith, is always hopeful, and endures through every circumstance.

Prophecy and speaking in tongues in unknown languages and special knowledge will become useless. But love will last forever! Now our knowledge is partial and incomplete, and even the gift of prophecy reveals only part of the whole picture! But when the time of perfection comes, these partial thing will become useless.

When I was a child, I spoke and thought and reasoned as a child. But when I grew up, I put away childish things. Now we see things imperfectly, like puzzling reflections in a mirror, but then we will see everything with perfect clarity. All that I know is partial and incomplete, but then I will know everything completely, just as God now knows me completely.

Spiritual Benefits of a God-Centered Paradigm

Three things will last forever—faith, hope, and love—and the greatest of these is love.

I decided to put in the whole chapter of 1 Corinthians 13, because it gives great context and emphasizes the importance of love. You are to have a godly kind of love in the manner you live your life. You are to love God with all your heart, soul, and mind. Then you are to love your neighbors as yourself.

That implies that you are also to love yourself, so that you know how to love your neighbors. But God wants you to take your love to another level; as in Matthew 5:44, where it says you are to love and pray for your enemies. Then in John 15:13 it states that no greater love than this is to lay down one's life for his friends, just as Christ laid down His life to save us.

Love is the supreme fruit of the Spirit. I hope and pray that your basket of fruit is huge, beautiful, and delicious.

Galatians 5:14 NLT

For the whole law can be summed up in this one command: 'Love your neighbor as yourself.'

I agape you!

Chapter 7
Paradigms in the Bible

Ephesians 1:16-19

I have not stopped thanking God for you. I pray for you constantly, asking God, the glorious Father of our Lord Jesus Christ, to give you spiritual wisdom and insight so that you might grow in your knowledge of God. I pray that your hearts will be flooded with light so that you can understand the confident hope he has given those he called—his holy people who are his rich and glorious inheritance. I also pray that you will understand the incredible greatness of God's power for us who believe him.

At first thought you might think: What do paradigms have to do with the Bible? But, there are actually many examples of paradigms in the Bible. There are paradigms involving individuals, groups of people, and nations. A country or culture (as I discussed in Chapter 1) has a paradigm of its own. A certain group of people can have similar views, perceptions, beliefs, or paradigms. I am going to cover some examples of paradigms involving well known stories in the Bible. I hope that looking at these stories from a different perspective will be entertaining and informative.

Twelve Scouts Explore Canaan

This story is found in Numbers Chapters 13 and 14 in the Old Testament. Moses has led the Israelites out of bondage in Egypt. They are on their way to the land promised to them by God. The Lord told Moses to send out men to explore the land of Canaan. He was to send one leader from each of the tribes of Israel. These men were not just random men from each tribe, but they were a leader in the tribe. So, they should be the most spiritually mature and knowledgeable people of Israel.

When they reached the valley of Eshcol (which means *cluster*), they cut down a single cluster of grapes. It was so large they had to carry it on a pole between two men. They also brought back pomegranates and figs. They had explored the land of Canaan for forty days.

When returning to Moses, Aaron, and the whole community of Israel, they gave a report to everyone. They showed them the fruit they brought back with them. They reported that the land was bountiful—a land flowing with milk and honey. But, the people living there were strong and powerful. They lived in large towns that were well fortified. They saw giant men there that made them feel like grasshoppers next to them. These giants thought that they were small and weak. The scouts reported that we cannot go up against them, as they will devour us.

But Caleb who was one of the scouts who stood up and tried to reassure and quiet the people. He said, "Let us go at once to conquer the land, as we can win."

The whole of Israel began weeping and crying all night. They eventually rose up against Moses and Aaron. They complained that they should have stayed and died in Egypt or in the wilderness. Why is the Lord taking us to this land, only to have us die in battle? They cried out that their children and wives would be taken as plunder. The people of Israel said, "Let's choose a new leader and go back to Egypt!"

Here are God's chosen people, whom He has just freed from Egypt. They had been a first-hand witness to God's power while they were in Egypt. They saw the Nile River turn red with blood. They were witnesses to the infestations of lice and fleas. They saw the Egyptian's livestock die. There were boils covering the men and animals. They saw a thunderstorm of hail and fire. The locusts came, which was followed by three days of darkness. They heard the cries of the mothers who lost their firstborn sons. The people of Israel saw God's power firsthand.

They were freed from Egypt, but then they were being chased down by the Egyptian army to be destroyed. The Israelites were trapped up against the banks of the Red Sea. Then Moses, through the power of God, parted the sea. What a sight that must have been to witness!

There is some controversy about whether the people of Israel crossed the Red Sea or the Persian Gulf, which is sometimes called the Arabian Gulf. The Persian Gulf is 615 miles long; the width varies from two hundred miles across to thirty-five miles across at the Strait of Hormuz. The Persian Gulf is much shallower than the Red Sea, with a maximum depth of about three hundred feet.

Ron Wyatt, who has been searching for the location of the crossing of Israel, believes that he has found the site of the crossing in the Persian Gulf at Nuweiba. The Nuweiba beach is large enough to hold the nearly 2.5 million Israelites. Ron Wyatt has found remains of chariots on the bottom of the sea in this area.

Other people believe they crossed at the Strait of Hormuz, which is only thirty-five miles wide and shallow. There is a ridge located there that the people of Israel could have used.

It is amazing to me that all these researchers are trying to find ways to make the crossing more plausible. The water is shallower or the width is shorter. The researchers look for areas on the sea floor, where it would be possible for the people to cross. They fail to see that if God created this whole universe, then it would be simple to divide the water of the

Red Sea or Persian Gulf. For God, it would simply be saying that the water should part and it would happen, no matter the location!

The Red Sea is about fourteen hundred miles long and averages about two hundred miles in width. The Red Sea (in the area that it is believed to have been the site of the crossing) reaches to a depth over 2,600 feet deep. The sides of the water where it was parted could have been nearly 3,000 feet high. Other locations proposed have a depth of nearly 5,000 feet deep. Can you imagine walking across the bottom of the Red Sea with the sides of the water twice as high as the Empire State building! The water is described in the Bible as a straight wall of water.

Not only that—the bottom of the sea floor was dry. That seems unbelievable in itself. And the floor of the sea had to be smoothed out, in order for them to traverse the bottom. Normally, there would be drop offs, reefs, and crevices which would keep them from crossing. God not only parted the water, but He prepared a dry road for them as well.

The Red Sea parting is an amazing story. The producer of the movie *The Ten Commandments*, Cecil B. DeMille, missed a huge opportunity. In the movie you see the people of Israel running down into the floor of the Red Sea—and just a minute later they are exiting on the other side. There were approximately two and one half million people leaving Egypt. The Red Sea is two hundred miles across. They would be lucky to travel fifteen miles a day. It may have taken them two weeks to cross the Red Sea!

Can you imagine camping on the floor of the Red Sea, with a wall of water reaching up as high as a tall skyscraper? You could be camping next to the wall of water with your campfire burning and have this unbelievable aquarium right next to you. The wall of this aquarium would be the largest ever built. There could be a huge 35 foot whale shark swimming right next to you, while you are cooking your dinner. The beautiful coral formations and multicolored fish would be a tremendous sight. It would be a pretty eerie feeling, sitting there observing it all. In fact, it is impossible to describe the immensity of it.

There are people who stand in line to go through the aquarium in Atlanta. You are on a moving walkway that goes under water that is just 40 feet deep. The scene as they are traversing the Red Sea would have been awesome. Hollywood could have made the parting of the Red Sea a magnificent event. Remember the scenery in the movie *Avatar* which was awe inspiring. The producers of *The Ten Commandments* missed a chance to make movie history. Although they still would have failed to capture the beauty, as seen by one who had actually been there.

Two weeks later, the people of Israel exit the Red Sea on the other side. What do you think the army of Egypt was thinking? They had witnessed all the miracles that God performed. I am sure many of them had lost a firstborn son. As they are camping overnight inside the parting of the Red Sea, are they worried about what might happen next? Are they mad because they had lost a son and can't wait to catch up to the Israelites? They should have been worried. God finished off the Egyptian army by closing the Red Sea over them.

The Israelites should have been overwhelmed with the power and love of God—but witnessing the power of God did not end there. The Lord appeared to the Israelites every day. He led them as a pillar of a cloud during the day and a pillar of fire at night. They saw His presence 24/7. They witnessed all these things and still did not understand the power of God. Their paradigms were very skewed, in view of what they had experienced. They should have had no fear or worries about following their God. Just three days after exiting the Red Sea, they started complaining to Moses about what was going to happen to them. One month after leaving Egypt, their complaints grew stronger. Exodus 16:3 says, *If only the Lord had killed us back in Egypt.*

After experiencing all the things recorded in the Bible and having God's presence in front of them every day, they still failed to perceive, see, or understand God's love and power. That is still true today. People are too busy and don't take the time to have a God-centered paradigm.

Except for the two scouts, Caleb and Joshua, the other leaders of the tribes of Israel failed to understand their circumstances. Even after witnessing God's power, they were afraid to follow His will. The scouts were timid and scared. They said that they had explored a wonderful land, but it was too dangerous and the people there were too big and strong. Only Caleb and Joshua said that if God was pleased with them, He would bring them safely into the land and give it to them. They said that God would make the people of Canaan a helpless prey, because the Lord is with us. But still the people of Israel were afraid and unhappy. Their memories were very short lived.

Exodus 14:31 NLT

When the people of Israel saw the mighty power that the Lord unleashed against the Egyptians, they were filled with awe before him. They put their faith in the Lord and his servant Moses.

Like many of us, you forget quickly. You are afraid to trust God completely.

The Lord became very upset with Israelites for their failure to believe in Him and for their rebelling against Him. Moses pleaded for mercy. The people of Israel were punished. God decreed that none of them over age twenty would enter the land of Canaan, except for Caleb and Joshua.

The ten scouts who did not trust in the Lord, or did not have a paradigm that recognized God as their Lord and Creator, were struck dead with a plague. Because of the Israelites paradigm they were banned from the Promised Land and spent forty years in the desert.

Gideon Becomes Israel's Judge

This story is found in Judges Chapter 6. Israel was reduced to starvation by Midianites continually destroying their crops. The Israelites cried to the Lord for help. The Israelites had begun to worship the gods of the Amorites. Even Gideon's father had built an altar to Baal.

The angel of the Lord comes to Gideon and greets him as a mighty hero. The angel tells Gideon that the Lord will be with him. Gideon questioned the angel, "If the Lord is with us, why has this happened to us? Why has the Lord abandoned us and handed us over to the Midianites?"

Then the Lord told Gideon to go with the strength that he has and rescue Israel from the Midianites. "I am sending you, Gideon," says the Lord. Gideon asks the Lord, "How can I rescue Israel? My clan is the weakest in the whole tribe of Manasseh. I am the least in my entire family." The Lord replied that He would be with him.

With his present knowledge or paradigm, Gideon did not understand how God could use lowly little him. Gideon asked for a sign. He needed reassurance or a change in his paradigm. Gideon prepared a sacrifice for God. The angel of God told him to place the meat and unleavened bread on a rock. He was instructed to pour the broth over it. The angel touched the meat and bread with the tip of his staff and a fire flamed up from the rock and consumed all the sacrifice.

Gideon built an altar to the Lord on that spot. He tore down the Baal altar and built an altar to God. Gideon was then called Jerubbaal which means *let Baal defend himself*. Soon after, the armies of the Midian, Amalek, and the people of the east formed an alliance against Israel. But Gideon needed more proof that God was with him. He still wasn't totally connected to God and asked for more evidence from Him.

Gideon placed a wool fleece on the threshing floor. If God was with him, the fleece would be wet with dew, but the ground around it would be dry. Gideon found it to be true. Like many of us, Gideon still needed more convincing and reassurance. He then asked that the fleece remain dry and the ground around it be wet. The next morning the fleece was dry and the ground was wet. Now Gideon was ready to lead the army! His paradigm had shifted. It is a shame that God has to keep proving Himself to us; but He is willing to do so, because of the love He has for us.

Because God wanted to try and change the Israelites' paradigm, he told Gideon that he had too many warriors. (It might allow the Israelites to think that through their own strength, they defeated the armies of Midian.) So, Gideon was instructed to tell the people of his army that if anyone was timid or afraid, they should go home. God was giving them another test of faith and altering their paradigms. Twenty-two thousand men went home.

But God wasn't done yet, God wanted to make an even bigger impression on the people of Israel. Sometimes people need to see some shock and awe to get the message. God told Gideon there were still too many in Gideon's now small army. So, God told Gideon that only the men who drank water from the stream with their hands would be allowed to stay for the battle. Three hundred men drank water with their hands. Now, we are getting down to bare bones level of men.

Just after midnight, Gideon and his three hundred men surrounded the army of Midian. There were so many men. It was like they were the grains of sand on a beach. There were too many to count. Following God's instruction, the three hundred men surrounded the camp and sounded their ram's horns and broke their jars. They held the blazing torches in their left hands and the horns in their right hands. They shouted, "A sword for the Lord and for Gideon." The warriors in the camp became confused. They began to fight and kill each other. Those that were not killed fled.

Initially Gideon did not trust God. He needed proof that God was with him. God also wanted to change the paradigms of the Israelites and show them that the victory over the army of Midian was due to Him. God was trying to impress upon the Israelites who He is. For a time, I am sure that the people of Israel realized who God was and had a new paradigm.

But, your paradigms can shift. Depending on what you are doing and what information you are putting into your mind, your paradigm can change.

David and Goliath

This story is found in 1 Samuel Chapter 17. The Philistines and the Israelites gathered their armies for battle, on hillsides on opposite sides of the valley of Elah. Goliath was the Philistine champion from Gath. He came out of the Philistine ranks to face the army of Israel. He was over nine feet tall! He wore a large bronze helmet. His bronze coat of mail weighed 125 pounds. He also wore bronze leg armor. He carried a bronze javelin on his shoulder. The tip of his spear was an iron spearhead that weighed fifteen pounds. His armor bearer walked ahead of him carrying the shield.

Goliath would shout a taunt to the Israelites saying, "Choose one man to come down here and fight me! If he kills me, then we will be your slaves. But if I kill him, you will be our slaves! I defy the armies of Israel today! Send me a man who will fight me!"

When Saul and his army heard this, they were terrified! Goliath taunted them for forty days each morning and evening. Isn't it interesting that these two armies got up every day, put on their battle gear, looked at other, and decided not to fight—only to get up the next day and do the same thing again?

David was the youngest son of Jesse, an Ephrathite from Bethlehem. Jesse's oldest sons were with Saul's army. David would travel back and forth, so he could help his father tend the sheep. David was in camp as the Israelite army was headed for the battlefield. The two sides were facing each other again. Goliath came out to give his usual performance. David asked the soldiers, "What will a man get for killing Goliath and ending his defiance of Israel? Who is this pagan Philistine anyway? How is he allowed to defy the armies of the living God?" Saul had offered a huge reward for anyone who would kill Goliath.

Look at the difference in David's paradigm versus that of the whole army of Israel. His faith in God allowed him to see Goliath with different eyes or God-centered eyes. He didn't see this huge unbeatable warrior as everyone else. He just saw someone who was disrespecting God's people. He was someone who could be easily defeated with God's help.

Hearing that David was asking questions about Goliath, his oldest brother approached him. He asked him what he was doing there, because he should be tending the sheep. David's questioning was reported to King Saul and He was escorted to meet with the king. David told Saul—no sweat, a piece of cake, he would fight Goliath. Saul's reply was that it was impossible, as he was only a boy. Saul was sure that he had no chance. (This is Saul's paradigm.) David persisted. He said that he had killed lions and bears while tending sheep. He could do the same thing to this pagan Philistine Goliath, for he had defied the armies of the living God! Since no one in forty days had stepped forward to volunteer, Saul finally agreed. Saul gave David permission to go ahead.

David did not want to use any armor. He wouldn't need any armor, as God was in his paradigm. He picked up five smooth stones from a stream and put them in his shepherd's bag. He was armed with only his shepherd's staff and sling, as he started across the valley. What did that have to look like, as he approached this mountain of man in front of him? The scene had to be unreal, as these two armies watched.

You have three paradigms involved with this battle. The Philistine army was positive that no one could defeat their champion. When they saw this shepherd boy with no armor or sword, they probably couldn't believe their eyes. What are the Israelites thinking? This fight was going to last only a second or two. (Which happens to be correct. It's just not the way they were imagining.)

The Israelite army was baffled, as well. We are sending this unarmed young boy to fight this giant. They resign themselves to defeat. They are going to be the slaves of the Philistines!

Only David had the correct paradigm. He knew that this giant was no match for his God. He was confident that, through the power of God, he would be victorious. Now imagine how everyone's paradigm plays out.

Goliath couldn't believe what he saw! The Israelite army was sending out a boy. What are they thinking? "Am I a dog," he roared at David, "that you come at me with a stick?" And he cursed David by the names of his gods. "Come over here, and I'll give your flesh to the birds and wild animals!" Goliath yelled.

The only person who had the correct paradigm was David. He was full of confidence, because his paradigm was centered on God. Look what David replies back to Goliath's taunts.

"You come to me with sword, spear, and javelin, but I come to you in the name of the Lord of Heaven's Armies—the God of the armies of Israel, whom you have defied. Today the Lord will conquer you, and I will kill you and cut off your head. And I will give the dead bodies of your men to the birds and wild animals, and the whole world will know that there is a God in Israel! And everyone assembled here will know that the Lord rescues His people, but not with a sword and spear. This is the Lord's battle, and He will give you to us!"

Goliath moved forward to attack David. David quickly ran out to meet him. He took a stone from his shepherd's bag and threw it at Goliath with his sling. He hit Goliath right in the middle of his forehead. The stone sank deep into his forehead. Goliath stumbled and fell face done on the ground.

(Someone that big may have had acromegaly, which is an over production of growth hormone. People who have this have very prominent foreheads with very thick frontal bones.)

David's shot had to be a perfect strike. It also had to be a very powerful strike, in order to put down Goliath. But through the power of God, no problem. David ran over and pulled Goliath's sword from its sheath. He used it to kill him and cut off his head.

David was brought before King Saul who asked him who his father was? David replied, "His name is Jesse, and we live in Bethlehem." The place where the most important event in the history of mankind would occur many years later.

David had a God-centered paradigm!

Elisha and the Arameans

This story is found in 2 Kings Chapter 6. The King of Aram was very upset with Elisha, because he was able to tell the King of Israel every move that he (the King of Aram) would plan in his war with Israel. The King of Aram decided that he was going to capture Elisha. They found out that Elisha was in Dothan. One night the King of Aram sent his troops of many chariots and horses to seize him. The troops surrounded the house where Elisha was staying.

When the servant of Elisha woke up early that morning, he went outside and saw that there were soldiers, horses, and chariots everywhere. The servant ran back inside and told Elisha that they were surrounded by a large army! Elisha tells his servant not to be afraid! He says, "For there are more on our side than on theirs!" (Evidently, Elisha was able to see into the spiritual realm, but not his servant.)

Then Elisha prayed, "O Lord, open his eyes and let him see!" The Lord opened the servant's eyes. When he looked up, he saw that the hillside around them was filled with horses and chariots of fire. By the power of God, the servant had a new paradigm. God had allowed his eyes to see into a different realm.

Like I discussed in the earlier chapters, your paradigm determines what you see, perceive, and understand. God allowed him to see things differently. You have that same ability to change your paradigm. You can look at your surrounding environment and perceive things in a completely different manner.

Saul's Conversion

Saul's conversion is found in Acts Chapter 9. You have also heard the term *paradigm shift*. Paradigm shift is a dramatic change from one set of parameters to a new set of parameters, such as the invention of the quartz watch. This story is about a tremendous paradigm shift.

Saul was present at the stoning of Stephen. Saul was uttering threats with every breath that he took and was eager to kill the Lord's followers. So he went to the high priest. He requested letters be addressed to the synagogues in Damascus, asking for their cooperation in the arrest of any followers of the Way that he found there. He wanted to bring them back to Jerusalem for trial.

As he was approaching Damascus on his mission, a light from heaven suddenly shined down. He fell to the ground and heard a voice saying, "Saul! Saul! Why are you persecuting me?" Saul replied, "Who are you, Lord?" Saul picked himself up off the ground, but when he opened his eyes, he was blind. So his companions had to lead him by the hand the rest of the way to Damascus. He remained there blind for three days, not eating or drinking. God sent a believer named Ananias to heal him. When Ananias found Saul, he laid his hands on him and said, "Brother Saul, the Lord Jesus, who appeared to you on the road, has sent me—so that you might regain your sight and be filled with the Holy Spirit."

Saul instantly regained his sight and got up. Saul was baptized and became a follower of Christ. Saul stayed with the believers in Damascus for a several days. He immediately began preaching about Jesus in the synagogues, that Jesus is indeed the Son of God. All who heard him were amazed. How can this be? Isn't this the same man who caused tremendous devastation to the followers of Jesus in Jerusalem?

Saul is now Paul. What a paradigm shift that was. He went from being a zealot persecutor of the followers of Jesus to the most fervent follower of Jesus. That is what the power of the Holy Spirit can do. You can be totally transformed, a new creature, and new paradigm.

There are many verses in the Bible that relate to paradigms and perceptions. The book of Isaiah has several verses about the people of Israel not listening or recognizing God in their lives. Many of the verses are telling about the coming of Jesus.

Isaiah 29:17-19 NLT

Soon—and it will not be very long—the forests of Lebanon will become a fertile land, and the fertile field will yield bountiful crops. In that day the deaf will hear words read from a book, and the blind will see through the gloom and darkness. The humble will be filled with fresh joy from the Lord. The poor will rejoice in the Holy One of Israel.

Isaiah 32:1-3 NLT

Look, a righteous king is coming! And honest princes will rule under him. Each one will be like a shelter from the wind and a refuge from the storm, like streams of water in the desert and the shadow of a great rock in a parched land. Then everyone who has eyes will be able to see the truth, and everyone who has ears will be able to hear it.

Isaiah 35:5 NLT

In that day those who cannot hear will hear the words of a book. And the eyes of the blind will see out of the darkness.

Isaiah 42:16, 18-20, 23 NLT

I will lead the blind by a way that they do not know. I will lead them in paths they do not know. I will turn darkness into light in front of them. And I will make the bad places smooth. These are the things I will do and I will not leave them. Listen, you who are deaf! Look and see, you blind! Who is blind as my own people, my servant? Who is as deaf as my messenger? Who is as blind as my chosen people, the servant of the Lord? You see and recognize what is right but refuse to act on it. You hear with your ears, but you don't really listen. Who will hear these lessons from the past and see the ruin that awaits you in the future?

Isaiah 43:8 NLT

Bring out the people who are blind, even though they have eyes, and those who cannot hear, even though they have ears.

Isaiah 44:18-20 NLT

Such stupidity and ignorance! Their eyes are closed, and they cannot see. Their minds are shut, and they cannot think. The person who made the idol never stops to reflect, Why, it's just a block of wood! I burned half of it for heat and used it to bake my bread and roast my meat. How can the rest of it be a God? Should I bow down to worship a piece of wood? The poor, deluded fool feeds on ashes. He trusts something that can't help him at all. Ye he cannot bring himself to ask, "Is this idol that I'm holding in my hand a lie?"

Jeremiah 5:20-24 NLT

Make this announcement to Israel, and say this to Judah: Listen, you foolish and senseless people, with eyes that do not see and ears that do not hear. Have you no respect for me? Why don't you tremble in my presence? I, the Lord, define the ocean's sandy shoreline as an everlasting boundary that the waters cannot cross. The waves mat toss and roar, but they can never pass the boundaries I set. But my people have stubborn and rebellious hearts. They have turned away and abandoned me. They do not say from the heart, Let us live in awe of the Lord our God, for he gives us rain each spring and fall, assuring us of a harvest when the time is right.

Matthew 13:10-16 NLT

His disciples came and asked him, Why do you use parables when you talk to the people? He replied, You are permitted to understand the secrets of the Kingdom of Heaven, but others are not. To those who listen to my teaching, more understanding will be given, and they will have an abundance of knowledge. But for those who are not listening, even what little understanding they have will be taken away from them. That is why I use parables, For they look, but they don't really see. They hear, but they don't really listen or understand. This fulfills the prophecy of Isaiah that says, When you hear what I say, you will not understand. When you see what I do, you will not comprehend. For the hearts of these people are hardened, and their ears cannot hear, and they have closed their eyes—so their eyes cannot see, and their ears cannot hear, and their hearts cannot understand, and they cannot turn to me and let me heal them. But blessed are your eyes, because they see; and your ears, because they hear. I tell you the truth, many prophets and righteous people longed to see what you see, but they didn't see it. And they longed to hear what you hear, but they didn't hear it.

Matthew 23:24-25 NLT

Blind guides! You strain your water so that you won't accidentally swallow a gnat, but you swallow a camel! What sorrow awaits you teachers of religious law and you Pharisees. Hypocrites! For you are so careful to clean the outside of the cup and the dish, but inside you are filthy—full of greed and self-indulgence! You blind Pharisee!

Mark 8:14-21 NLT

But the disciples had forgotten to bring any food. They only had one loaf of bread with them in the boat. As they were crossing the lake, Jesus warned them, "Watch out! Beware of the yeast of the Pharisees and of Herod." As they began to argue with each other because they hadn't brought any bread, Jesus knew what they were saying, so he said, "Why are you arguing about having no bread? Don't you know or understand even yet? Are your hearts too hard to take it in? You have eyes—can't you see? You have ears—can't you hear? Don't you remember anything at all? When I fed the 5,000 with five loaves of bread, how many baskets of leftovers did you pick up afterward?" "Twelve," they said. "And when I fed the 4,000 with seven loaves, how many large baskets of leftovers did you pick up?" "Seven," they said. "Don't you understand yet?" he asked them.

Luke 10:21-23 NLT

At that same time Jesus was filled with the Holy Spirit, and he said, "O Father, Lord of heaven and earth, thank you for hiding these things from those who think themselves wise and clever, and for revealing them to the childlike. Yes, Father, it pleased you to do it this way." My Father has entrusted everything to me. No one truly knows the Son except the Father, and no one truly knows the Father except the Son and those to whom the Son choses to reveal him. Then when they were alone, he turned to the disciples and said, "Blessed are the eyes that see what you have seen. I tell you, many prophets and kings longed to see what you see, but they didn't see it. And they longed to hear what you hear, but they didn't hear it."

John 9:35-41 NLT

When Jesus heard what had happened, he found the man and sked, "Do you believe in the Son of Man?" the man answered, "Who is he, sir? I want to believe in him." "You have seen him," Jesus said, "and he is speaking to you!" 'Yes, Lord, I believe!" the man said. And he worshiped Jesus. The Jesus told him, "I entered this world to render judgement—to give sight to the blind and to show those who think they see that they are blind." Some Pharisees who were standing nearby heard him and asked, "Are you saying we're blind?" "If you were blind, you wouldn't be guilty," Jesus replied. "But you remain guilty because you claim you can see."

2 Corinthians 4:1-4 NLT

Therefore, since God in his mercy has given us this new way, we never give up. We reject all shameful deeds and underhanded methods. We don't try to trick anyone or distort the word of God. We tell the truth before God, and all who are honest know this. If the Good News we preach is hidden behind a veil, it is hidden only from people who are perishing. Satan, who is the god of this world, has blinded the minds of those who don't believe. They are unable to see the glorious light of the Good News. They don't understand this message about the glory of Christ, who is the exact likeness of God.

There are many more Bible verses about not seeing, perceiving, or hearing because their paradigms were not tuned into or centered on God.

Satan fools many people as he is the great deceiver. The anti-Christ will do the same thing when he comes. The anti-Christ will fool many people, because people will fail to perceive what is before them.

The most incredible example of a paradigm in the Bible is about Jesus.

The Jewish people had been waiting for the Messiah. It had been 400 years since the last prophet Malachi. In Malachi chapter 3, he tells of the coming of the Lord. There are many Bibles verses in the Old Testament that tell of the coming of Jesus or the Messiah. In the New Testament, the people of Israel find themselves under the rule of another nation. Just like all the times in the past, they had turned away from God. This time it was the Roman Empire. They were tired of the oppression from the Romans, and they were focused on the predicted coming of the Messiah.

Even though the Old Testament is full of verses describing the Messiah, it didn't matter. They had their own beliefs or paradigm about who the Messiah was going to be. They were looking for another Moses to use God's power to get rid of the Romans. Or maybe they were watching for a person like Samson, who slew one thousand Philistines with the jawbone of a donkey. Maybe someone like the great King David. At least he was going to be this big, strong, warrior who would nearly single-handedly run the Romans out of town. He would be their powerful king of kings.

They were very well aware of all the Old Testament prophecies. I am sure it was taught and discussed routinely at their synagogue. You know that the Pharisees and Sadducees knew the Scriptures thoroughly, but they still couldn't believe that their Messiah was going to be born in a shed or barn.

Jesus would appear to be an illegitimate son, as Joseph and Mary were not married yet. The angel appeared to Joseph to let him know about the virgin birth of Jesus—that Jesus would be clothed in swaddling clothes, instead of silk pajamas. He would be born to a blue-collar family, not royalty. He had no money or wealth. He would spend his early life as a lowly carpenter, not a soldier in training or in a beautiful palace. This man was going to preach love. He was even going to tell you to love your enemies. They were to love the Romans!! How crazy is that? He had no sword, no armor, and no army to lead the Jewish people into to battle with the Romans. He rode into main street Jerusalem on a donkey!

There was the Son of God right in front of their face. He had fulfilled all the Old Testament prophecies about the Messiah. He performed all kinds of miracles. He even brought people back from the dead. Lazarus had been dead for four days. His body would have been decomposing in that tomb, but he came alive—fresh as a daisy. But in the end, they would crucify the Messiah, the Son of God!

Let's take a look at an example where they refused to see the Son of God who was right in front of them. What a closed mind and paradigm these people had in the New Testament. But today, is it any different?

In John Chapter 9 there is a story about Jesus healing a man who was blind from birth. It is interesting how he healed the blind man. He could have just said, "See" and the man would have gained his vision. Instead, he spits on the ground, made some mud with the saliva, and put it on the man's eyes. Jesus told him to go to the pool of Siloam (this word means *sent*) and wash off the mud. He immediately washed off the mud and he could immediately see.

Maybe Jesus used the mud as a symbol of what God made us from. It is possible that Jesus was trying to give everyone a clue about who he was by sending him to the pool of Siloam. There is some evidence that the people of that time thought that saliva had some healing properties. So instead of just healing the man, he wanted people to look a little deeper into the miracle.

The man went home. His neighbors and people who knew him could not believe what they were seeing (no pun intended). The man they knew had been blind from birth. Some thought that maybe this man was someone who looked like the man they knew. But the man informed them that it was him. He told them that Jesus had healed him. They were so amazed that they took him to the Pharisees.

There was a problem—Jesus had healed him on the Sabbath. According to the law, no work of any kind is to be done on the Sabbath. The Pharisees asked him how he was healed. He told them the events of his healing. Some of the Pharisees were upset because Jesus had healed this man on the Sabbath. Others wondered how a sinner could perform such a miracle. They asked the man what he thought. He said that Jesus was a prophet.

The Pharisees did not want to believe that Jesus had healed this blind man, so now they were going to have an instant and mostly rigged trial. They send for the man's parents. The parents are questioned to make sure that he was really blind. They wanted the parents to tell them some story that they could believe about their son being cured. The parents confirmed their son was born blind and now could see. They were afraid of the Pharisees and refused to say anything more.

The Jewish leaders had already decreed that anyone who acknowledged Jesus as the Messiah would be banned from the synagogue. You would think that they would have supported Jesus, who had just performed a miracle on their son. Their son could be a productive member of society. He would be able to work now that he could see. They would no longer have to take care of him. But no, they were afraid.

The Pharisees were not going to let this go. They summoned the healed blind man back for a second round of questioning. Maybe, they could make him change his story. This time they got into a confrontation with the man. The Pharisees hurled insults at the man stating that he was a disciple of Jesus. They were all pious and mighty, because they were disciples of Moses. The healed blind man tells them that if this man were not from God, he could do none of the miracles he was performing. The Pharisees threw the man out. Court adjourned!! They didn't get the result they were looking for.

The evidence is obvious. It was verified that the man was born blind. They were able to examine him and see that he could see. Here was all this evidence, right before their very eyes, yet they refused or couldn't see or understand it. Because of their paradigm, their brains or minds were unable to see something obvious right in front of them.

There were no smoke or mirrors. Jesus is going to give the answer. Jesus hears that the Pharisees have thrown the man out. Jesus finds the man and asks him if he believes in the Son of Man. The healed blind man says that he does believe and worships Jesus.

Jesus tells him, "For judgment I have come into this world, so that the blind will see and those who see will become blind." The Pharisees who heard this asked Jesus if they were blind. Jesus said, "If you were blind, you would not be guilty of sin; but now that you claim you can see, your guilt remains."

The Pharisees had a bad paradigm. They were too into themselves, their lives, money, and prestige. They were not going to give up the good racket they were running. Eventually they realize that they must get rid of Jesus and decide to execute him. Other than telling the leaders of the Jewish people that they were wrong, He had nothing but love and compassion for everyone.

How did things change in a few days from Jesus riding into Jerusalem on a donkey to a glorious celebration to the people wanting him crucified? People can be easily influenced by a mob or group of people. The mind can be influenced or a paradigm changed quickly under the right circumstances.

The Pharisees and Sadducees were so afraid of Jesus that they wanted to make an example of Him. He couldn't come to them and tell about the Torah and God! So, they didn't just decide to execute him—they were going to do it in the most gruesome manner. The word *excruciating* comes from the word crucifying. The religious leaders pressured Pilot to execute Jesus. Pilot had Jesus scourged as a punishment. He thought it should be enough, as he wasn't sure he was guilty of anything. Pilate felt that if Jesus had been severely scourged and made to look humiliated, he could set him free. Scourging was called *verberatio* by the Romans. It was to not only inflict severe pain, but to humiliate the person as well. After the scourging, the Roman soldiers would taunt and make fun of their victims. The Romans did not invent scourging, but they were experts at performing it.

Jesus was flogged with a whip that was made of leather braids, with iron balls and/or sharp pieces of sheep bones attached to the leather straps. He was stripped of his clothing and was naked as they tied him to a post. He was flogged on his back, buttocks, and legs to a state of collapse or just short of death. There could be extensive blood loss leading to shock.

Pilate brought Jesus before the people with a crown of thorns and a mock robe. Pilate felt that if he did enough punishment and humiliated Jesus, the people would be satisfied. He would show Jesus as a broken down man who could be no one's King! But the Pharisees were not going to stop until Jesus was dead. Also, the people were riled up and were still not satisfied. Eventually, they got what they wanted and Jesus was crucified.

It was the Roman custom that the condemned man had to carry the cross bar of the cross from the flogging post to the crucifixion site outside the city. He would be naked. One of the Roman soldiers would carry a sign which had the condemned man's name and crime. This would later be attached to the top of the cross. Once they reached the site of the crucifixion, the person was given a bitter drink of wine mixed with gall (myrrh) as a mild pain reliever. Jesus was nailed to the cross with iron spikes five to seven inches long. The length of time a person would live on the cross varied widely, depending on the severity of the scourging. Death could occur within a few hours to as long as three to four days. Death could be hastened by breaking the legs below the knees. This would keep them from using their legs to help them breathe.

Jesus only lived a few hours due to the severe scourging he received. To make sure that a person was dead, a Roman soldier would thrust a spear through the right side of the chest. It appears that this is what happened to Jesus. The spear most likely penetrated his right thin-walled atrium. The fluid that came from the wound either came from fluid in his lungs or from fluid around his heart. The fluid was followed by blood. Jesus died to save the world from its sin.

How could the people of Israel kill a man who only taught love and compassion? They killed their own Messiah! They had been praying for four hundred years to God that he would send the Messiah to them. Look what their beliefs and perceptions allowed them to do.

Romans 1:20 NLT

For ever since the world was created, people have seen the earth and sky. Through everything God made, they can clearly see his invisible qualities— his eternal power and divine nature. So they have no excuse for not knowing God.

Even today, people are unable to see, hear, comprehend, or understand the gospel of Jesus Christ. Their paradigms and understanding don't allow them to see God or perceive His presence in this world. In Revelation Chapter 3, Jesus says that He is at the door knocking. Whoever hears him and lets Him in, He will have a relationship with them. The question is, do you hear Him knocking or is your paradigm keeping you from hearing it or understanding what it means? Satan, the secular world, and our sinful selves are trying to muffle the sound. They don't want you to hear it.

You need to be careful about what you decide to make of your paradigm—what information you put into it and how you process the information. Learn from the Bible what it says about believing and seeing.

God, Jesus, and the Holy Spirit are communicating to you the plans they have for your life. Make sure that your mind and paradigm are on the same wavelength as theirs.

Listen, see, and perceive, you don't want to miss what they are saying!

Chapter 8
The Holy Spirit or God's Presence on Earth

1 Corinthians 2:10 NLT
But it was to us that God revealed these things by his Spirit. For his Spirit searches out everything and shows us God's deep secrets.

God shows you His divine nature, love, attributes, compassion, instruction, and His sacrifice for you through the Holy Spirit. The Holy Spirit opens the infinite depth of God's mind and reveals to you the things you need to know about life and the world you live in. We worship a God in heaven with Jesus at His right hand. The Holy Spirit is God on earth. You are taught many things about Jesus and God, but the Holy Spirit is not discussed or taught about in many churches. You will find the Holy Spirit throughout the Bible. The Holy Spirit of the Old Testament and the New Testament has very similar roles. The Holy Spirit performs many of the same tasks or functions in both. The main difference is that after Adam and Eve in the Old Testament, the Holy Spirit was only present in people for endeavors that God has chosen them for—a specific task, function, or to complete a divine plan that God wanted accomplished. In many cases, once the task had been completed, the Holy Spirit left. After Pentecost, the Holy Spirit became available to everyone.

In the Bible, there are three ways you can have a relationship with the Holy Spirit. The first way is that the Holy Spirit is **with us**. The

Holy Spirit is everywhere. You can choose to listen to the Holy Spirit or you can choose not to listen to the Holy Spirit.

Revelation 3:20 NLT

Look, I stand at the door and knock. If you hear my voice and open the door, I will come in, and we will share a meal together as friends.

The second way is that the Holy Spirit will be **in you**. Once you accept Jesus Christ as your Lord and Savior, the Holy Spirit enters you. You begin your relationship with him.

John 14:17 NLT

He is the Holy Spirit, who leads into all truth. The world cannot receive him, because it isn't looking for him and doesn't recognize him. But you know him, because he lives with you now and later will be in you.

The third way is the Holy Spirit may **come upon you**.

Acts1:8 NLT

But you will receive power when the Holy Spirit comes upon you. And you will be my witness.

There are many instances in the Bible where people did amazing things through the power of the Holy Spirit.

Let's take a look at some of the references to the Holy Spirit beginning in the Old Testament. You will see the many characteristics and attributes of the Holy Spirit.

The Holy Spirit in the Old Testament

Many people feel that the Holy Spirit first appeared in the Bible in the New Testament or at Pentecost. The Holy Spirit actually appears in the Bible in Genesis. The Holy Spirit was directly involved with the creation of the world.

Genesis 1:2 NLT

The earth was formless and empty, and darkness covered the deep waters. And the Spirit of God was hovering over the surface of the waters.

The Holy Spirit was God's presence on Earth. The Holy Spirit is responsible for your life. The Holy Spirit gives life as described in Job.

Job 33:4 NLT

For the Spirit of God has made me,
and the breath of the Almighty gives me life.

The Holy Spirit is not only your source of life, but is also a teacher, guide, and instructor. The Holy Spirit evidently enjoyed walking around the Garden of Eden observing the beauty of His creation.

Genesis 3:8 NLT

When the cool evening breezes were blowing, the man and his wife heard the Lord God walking about in the garden.

God's Spirit was present on earth and had a direct relationship with Adam. After Adam and Eve sinned, the Spirit of God left the earth. After Adam and Eve sinned, He only became involved with certain leaders, judges, and prophets found in the Old Testament.

There are many places in the Bible where the Holy Spirit was involved with leaders, such Moses, David, Elisha, Elijah, and others. In some ways you can understand why the Jewish people kept turning away from God. They did not have the advantage of the Holy Spirit in their lives. They had great leaders and prophets who were filled with the Holy Spirit, but many times the people of Israel failed to listen to them. In the Old Testament, God chose the people of Israel as His people. But the people of Israel turned their backs on God and His Holy Spirit time after time.

Zechariah 7:11-12 NLT

Your ancestors refused to listen to this message. They stubbornly turned away and put their fingers in their ears to keep from hearing. They made their hearts as hard as stone, so they could not hear the instructions or the messages that the LORD of Heaven's Armies had sent them by his Spirit through the earlier prophets.

Nehemiah 9:30 NLT

In your love, you were patient with them for many years. You sent your Spirit, who warned them through the prophets. But still they wouldn't listen!

The Holy Spirit is part of the Triune God that God the Father has placed here on earth.

Let us go through some of the instances where the Holy Spirit worked in the lives of people in the Old Testament. After Adam came Noah.

Noah

Genesis 6:9 NLT

This is the account of Noah and his family. Noah was a righteous man, the only blameless person living on earth at the time, and he walked in close fellowship with God. Noah had an intimate relationship with the Holy Spirit of God. Through Noah, God saved the plants, animals, and mankind.

Abram or Abraham

Genesis 12

This chapter is where God called Abram. God told him that all the families of earth would be blessed through him. God chose Abram to be the father of His people. God communicated with Abram on a regular basis. God later changed Abram's name to Abraham and again made a covenant with him.

Abraham also had a visit from whom many people believe was Jesus, which is found in Genesis.

Genesis 14:18-20 NLT

And Melchizedek, the king of Salem and priest of God Most High, brought Abram some bread and wine. Melchizedek blessed Abram with this blessing: 'Blessed be Abram by God Most High, Creator of heaven and earth. And blessed be God Most High, who has defeated your enemies for you.' Then Abram gave Melchizedek a tenth of all the goods he had recovered.

Many people believe that Melchizedek was Jesus.

Abraham fathered a son at age 100, through the power of God. Finally, Abraham proved his faith in God when he was going to sacrifice his son to God. Eventually, God would do the same thing in sacrificing His Son on the cross for you and me. God's love for you is beyond your or my comprehension.

Joseph

As you know Joseph ends up in Egypt because his brothers sold him to the Ishmaelite traders. Through the power of the Holy Spirit, Joseph interprets the Pharaoh's dreams. Pharaoh says this in Genesis.

Genesis 41:38-39 NLT

So Pharaoh asked his officials, 'Can we find anyone else like this man so obviously filled with the spirit of God?' Then Pharaoh said to Joseph, 'Since God has revealed the meaning of the dreams to you, clearly no one else is as intelligent or wise as you are.'

Through the power of the Holy Spirit, Joseph was able to interpret Pharaoh's dreams and also had the gift of the knowledge.

Moses

There are many instances in the Old Testament where through the power of the Holy Spirit, Moses performed miraculous feats and miracles—the plagues, parting of the Red Sea, and others. God decided to give His spirit to seventy elders to help Moses with managing all the nation of Israel.

Numbers 11:16-17 NLT

Then the Lord said to Moses, 'Gather before me seventy men who are recognized as elders and leaders of Israel. Bring them to the Tabernacle to stand there with you. I will come down and talk to you there. I will take some of the Spirit that is upon you, and I will put the Spirit upon them also.'

So you can see that God chose the people who would receive His Spirit. As you can see, the Holy Spirit was not available to everyone in the Old Testament.

God chose Bezalel and Oholiab to receive the Holy Spirit.

Exodus 31:1-6 NLT

The Lord said to Moses, Look, I have specifically chosen Bezalel son of Uri, the grandson of Hur, of the tribe of Judah. I have filled him with the Spirit of God, giving him great wisdom, ability, and expertise in all kinds of crafts. He is a master craftsman, expert in working with gold, silver, and bronze. He is skilled in engraving and mounting gemstones and in carving wood. He is a master at every craft. And I have personally appointed Oholiab son of Ahisamach, of the tribe of Dan, to be his assistant. Moreover, I have given special skill to all the gifted craftsmen so they can make all the things I have commanded you to make:

God gave these men special skills to perform the work that God had commanded Moses to complete. God gives His people the skills they need to complete the plan or tasks that He has for each one of us.

Exodus 35:30-35 NLT

Then Moses told the people of Israel, The Lord has specifically chosen Bezalel son of Uri, grandson of Hur, of the tribe of Judah. The Lord has filled Bezalel with the Spirit of God, giving him great wisdom, ability, and expertise in all kinds of crafts. He is a master craftsman, expert in working with gold, silver, and bronze. He is skilled in engraving and mounting gemstones and in carving wood. He is a master at every craft. And the Lord has given both him and Oholiab son of Ahisamach, of the tribe of Dan, the ability to teach their skills to others. The Lord has given them special skills as engravers, designers, embroiderers in blue, purple, and scarlet thread on fine linen cloth, and weavers. They excel as craftsman and designers. God through his Spirit has given these two men many skills to performs tasks for God.

Joshua

Numbers 27:18, 22-23 NLT

The Lord replied, Take Joshua son of Nun, who has the Spirit in him, and lay your hands on him. So Moses did as the Lord commanded, He presented Joshua to Eleazar the priest and the whole community. Moses laid his hands on him and commissioned him to lead the people.

Joshua was filled with the Spirit of God as we saw when he returned from scouting Canaan.

Judges

In the book of Judges, it talks about men whom God chose to lead the people of Israel. God filled these men with His Spirit to give them the power and abilities to lead.

Judges 2:16-18 NLT

Then the Lord raised up judges to rescue the Israelites from their attackers. Yet Israel did not listen to their judges but prostituted themselves by worshipping other Gods. How quickly they turned from the path of their ancestors, who had walked in obedience to the Lord's commands. Whenever the Lord raised up a judge over Israel, he was with that judge

The Holy Spirit or God's Presence on Earth

and rescued the people from their enemies throughout the judge's lifetime.
For the Lord took pity on his people,
who were burdened by oppression and suffering.

The Lord raised up judges to rescue the Israelites from their attackers or enemies. Whenever the Lord raised up a judge over Israel, the Holy Spirit was with that judge. The Holy Spirit, through the judge, rescued the people from their enemies throughout the judge's lifetime. Unfortunately, they reverted back to sinning against God after the death of the judge. The people of Israel never kept their focus on their God for very long.

Othniel

Judges 3:9-10 NLT

But when the people of Israel cried out to the Lord for help, the Lord raised up a rescuer to save them. His name was Othniel, the son of Caleb's younger brother, Kenaz. The Spirit of the Lord came upon him, he became Israel's judge. He went to war against King Cushan-rishathaim of Aram, and the Lord gave Othniel victory over him. So Othniel became Israel's first judge who was filled with the Holy Spirit.

After each judge passed away, the people of Israel would go back to worshipping idols, such as Baal.

Here is a list of the judges in the Old Yestament who through the Holy Spirit led the Israelites. There was Ehud, Deborah, Gideon (Gideon is covered earlier in the book), Tola, Jair, Jephthah, Ibzan, Elon, Abdon, and then came Samson. One judge that you may not remember did a feat almost as amazing as Samson. Shamgar killed six hundred Philistines with an ox goad. The Holy Spirit can make us all powerful.

Samson

Judges 13:24-25 NLT

When her son was born, she named him Samson. And the Lord blessed him as he grew up. And the Spirit of the Lord began

> *to stir him while he lived in Mahaneh-dan,*
> *which is located between the towns of Zorah and Eshtaol.*

The angel of the Lord told Samson's mother that his hair was not to be cut as a sign of his dedication to God. Samson was attacked by a lion and the Spirit of the Lord came upon him and he ripped the lion's jaw apart with hands. Later he was given over to the Philistines by the men of Judah. They tied him up with new rope.

Judges 15:14-15 NLT

As Samson arrived at Lehi, the Philistines came shouting in triumph. But the Spirit of the Lord came powerfully upon Samson, and he snapped the ropes on his arms as if they were burnt strands of flax, and they fell from his wrists. Then he found the jawbone of a recently killed donkey. He picked it up and killed one thousand Philistines with it.

Again, the Holy Spirit provided Samson with super human strength. Samson met Delilah and succumbed to her beauty. The Philistines bribed her to find out the secret of Samson's strength. Through her charm, she finally finds out the answer and Samson is captured as he has lost his strength. He sinned against God. As they were making fun of Samson, they placed him between two pillars that held up the roof of the temple. Samson asked God for his strength back and he brought down the temple with his hands. He killed all the people in the temple.

Throughout the Old Testament, God's Holy Spirit filled the judges in the Bible.

Another group of people that the Holy Spirit guided were the Kings of Israel.

Saul

Saul was anointed King of Israel by Samuel.

1 Samuel 10:9-10 NLT

As Saul turned and started to leave, God gave him a new heart, and all Samuel's signs were fulfilled that day. When Saul and his servant arrived at Gibeah, they saw a group of prophets coming toward them. Then the Spirit of God came powerfully upon Saul, and he, too began to prophesy.

Saul had been anointed King of Israel by Samuel. He received the Spirit to help him be King of Israel. God later removed the Spirit from Saul and Saul began to falter as King.

David

1 Samuel 16:13

So David stood there among his brothers, Samuel took the flask of olive oil he had brought and anointed David with oil. And the Spirit of the Lord came powerfully upon David from that day on.

1 Samuel 18:28-30

When Saul realized that the Lord was with David and how much his daughter Michal loved him, Saul became even more afraid of him, and he remained David's enemy for the rest of his life. Every time the commanders of the Philistines attacked, David was more successful against them than all the rest of Saul's officers. So, David's name became very famous.

Through the power of the Holy Spirit David was successful in all his battles.

Solomon

1 Kings 3:10-14 NLT

The Lord was pleased that Solomon had asked for wisdom. So God replied, 'Because you have asked for wisdom in governing my people with justice and have not asked for a long life or wealth or the death of your enemies—I will give you what you ask for! I will give you a wise and understanding heart such as no one else has had or will ever have! And I will give you what you did not ask for—riches and fame! No other king in all the world will be compared to you for the rest of your life! And if you follow me and obey my decrees and my commands as your father, David, did, I will give you a long life.'

The Holy Spirit gave Solomon the things that God promised him.

The other group of people that the Holy Spirit used to promote God's will for the people of Israel were the prophets in the Old Testament. The prophets in the Bible are generally divided into major and minor prophets. The major prophets are Isaiah, Jeremiah, Ezekiel, and Daniel. The minor prophets are Hosea, Joel, Amos, Obadiah, Jonah, Micah, Nahum, Habakkuk, Zephaniah, and Malachi. There many other lesser known prophets, as well. God spoke to the people of Israel through His Holy Spirit-filled prophets.

Balaam

Balaam was one of the earlier prophets in the Old Testament who was blessed by the Holy Spirit.

Numbers 24:2 NLT

Then the Spirit of God came upon him.

Isaiah

Isaiah means the *Salvation of Jehovah;* which he was, the prophet of salvation. In Isaiah Chapter 6 is the call of his mission as a prophet of God.

Isaiah does say in Isaiah Chapter 48 that *the Sovereign Lord and his Spirit have sent me with this message.* In Chapter 61 he says, *The Spirit of the Lord is upon me, for the Lord has anointed me to bring good news to the poor.* In the New Testament Paul refers to Isaiah as being *led by the Holy Spirit.*

Acts 28:25 NLT

And after they had argued back and forth among themselves, they left with their final word from Paul: The Holy Spirit was right when he said to your ancestors through Isaiah the prophet

Jeremiah

Jeremiah was chosen to be a prophet of God before he was born!

Jeremiah 1:4-10 NLT

The Lord gave me this message: "I knew you before I formed you in your mother's womb. Before you were born I set you apart and appointed you as my prophet to the nations." "O Sovereign Lord," I said, "I can't speak for you! I'm too young!" The Lord replied, "Don't say, 'I'm too young,' for you must go wherever I send you and say whatever I tell you. And don't be afraid of the people, for I will be with you and will protect you. I, the Lord, have spoken!" Then the Lord reached out and touched my mouth and said, "Look, I have put my words in your mouth! Today I appoint you to stand up against nations and kingdoms. Some you must uproot and tear down, destroy and overthrow. Others you must build up and plant.

That's a pretty intimidating assignment for a young man, but anything is possible with the power of the Holy Spirit. The Lord gave him a new paradigm, perception, or God's way of seeing.

Jeremiah 1:11-14 NLT

Then the Lord said to me, "Look, Jeremiah! What do you see?" and I replied, "I see a branch from an almond tree." And the Lord said, "That's right, and it means that I am watching, and I will certainly carry out all my plans." Then the Lord spoke to me again and asked, "What do you see now?" And I relied, "I see a pot of boiling water, spilling down from the north." "Yes," the Lord said, "for terror from the north will boil out on the people of this land. Listen! I am calling the armies of the kingdoms of the north to come to Jerusalem. I, the Lord, have spoken!

Jeremiah now has the power of the Holy Spirit and a new paradigm. He is able to see things differently. Also, did you notice Jeremiah saw that it was a branch of an almond tree? God said that it means he was going to be watching. What are on the branches of an almond tree? Almonds, right! It has been described by many that we have eyes that are shaped like almonds. Jeremiah could see that there were all these almonds or eyes looking at him.

God was going to be carefully watching him and supporting him.

Ezekiel

Ezekiel 2:1-3 NLT

"Stand up, son of man," said the voice. "I want to speak with you." The Spirit came into me as he spoke, and set me on my feet. I listened carefully to his words. "Son of man," he said, "I am sending you to the nation of Israel, a rebellious nation that has rebelled against me. They and their ancestors have been rebelling against me to this very day."

Ezekiel 11:18-21 NLT

When the people return to their homeland, they will remove every trace of their vile images and detestable idols. And I will give them singleness of heart and put a new spirit within them. I will take away their stony, stubborn heart and give them a tender, responsive heart, so they will obey my decrees and regulations. Then they will truly be my people, and I will be their God. But as for those who long for vile images and detestable idols, I will repay them fully for their sins.

Ezekiel was enabled to do all his tasks as well through the Holy Spirit.

Daniel

You probably know about the many things that Daniel did, as told in the book of Daniel. Daniel had the Holy Spirit to rely on. The hungry lions did not attack and eat him when he was thrown into the lion's den. His companions were not burned in the fire that they were thrown into. It was known throughout Babylon that he was filled with the Spirit of his God.

Daniel 4:8-9 NLT

At last Daniel came in before me, and I told him the dream. (He was named Belteshazzar after my god, and the spirit of the holy gods is in him.) I said to him, "Belteshazzar, chief of the magicians, I know that the spirit of the holy gods is in you and that no mystery is too great for you to solve. Now tell me what my dream means."

Daniel 5:11 NLT

There is a man in your kingdom who has within him the spirit of the holy gods.

Elijah

Elijah first appears in the Old Testament in 1 Kings Chapter 17.

Now Elijah, who was from Tishbe in Gilead, told King Ahab, "As surely as the Lord, the God of Israel, lives—the God I serve—there will be no dew or rain during the next few years until I give the word.

1 Kings 18:46 NLT

And soon the sky was black with clouds. A heavy wind brought a terrific rainstorm, and Ahab left quickly for Jezreel. Then the Lord gave special strength to Elijah. He tucked his cloak into his belt and ran ahead of Ahab's chariot all the way to the entrance of Jezreel.

Now tucking in a cloak into a belt and then running isn't the most efficient uniform to have on when running, especially a long distance. With the strength of the Holy Spirit, Elijah was able to run as fast as horses pulling a chariot! That would be a gold medal performance in the Olympics in any race! Can you imagine what King Ahab was thinking as he is fleeing from the storm and this man of God is running ahead of his chariot the whole way?

2 Kings 2:11-12 NLT

As they were walking along and talking, suddenly a chariot of fire appeared, drawn by horses of fire. It drove between the two men, separating them, and Elijah was carried by a whirlwind into heaven. Elisha saw it and cried out, "My father! My father! I see the chariots and charioteers of Israel!"

So, Elijah was taken to heaven without dying. Enoch is the only other person to have been taken to heaven without dying. Both were strong believers and followers of God.

Elisha

1 Kings 19:19-21 NLT

So Elijah went and found Elisha son of Shaphat plowing a field. There were twelve teams of oxen in the field, and Elisha was plowing with the twelfth team. Elijah went over to him and threw his cloak across his shoulders and then walked away. Elisha left the oxen standing there, ran after Elijah, and said to him, "First let me go and kiss my father and mother good-bye, and then I will go with you!"

The casting of his cloak or mantle is a symbol of Elijah adopting him. Since Elisha understood what it was related to, he probably received the Holy Spirit at the same time.

2 Kings 2:9-10 NLT

When they came to the other side, Elijah said to Elisha, "Tell me what I can do for you before I am taken away." And Elisha replied, "Please let me inherit a double share of your spirit and become your successor." "You have asked a difficult thing," Elijah replied, "If you see me when I am taken from you, then you will get your request.

So, Elisha received the Holy Spirit and became Elijah successor.

Zechariah

2 Chronicles 24:20 NLT

Then the Spirit came upon Zechariah son of Jehoiada the priest.

Micah

Micah 3:8 NLT

But as for me, I am filled with power—with the Spirit of the Lord. I am filled with justice and strength to boldly declare Israel's sin and rebellion.

As you can see there are many references to the Holy Spirit in the Old Testament. There are many more recordings of the Holy Spirit in the Old Testament than I covered here. God uses His Spirit to interact with people on earth. The people of Israel in the Old Testament lived by the laws given by God to Moses.

It isn't until Pentecost, that God's people would live under a new covenant and a new relationship. The Holy Spirit would become available to anyone who believes in Christ Jesus as their Savior. God again becomes intimately involved with His creation as His Spirit and man's spirit connect. The Old Testament ends open-ended with the foretelling of the coming of the Messiah and the Holy Spirit being more involved in the daily lives of many more people. There would be a new community of faithful followers of God.

The Holy Spirit in the New Testament

The Holy Spirit comes to earth on a full time basis in the New Testament. Man is just flesh and cannot enter the Kingdom of Heaven. God sends the Holy Spirit, so man can enter the Kingdom of Heaven. Nicodemus comes to Jesus to ask him questions. Jesus tells him what is required to enter the Kingdom of Heaven. Nicodemus does not understand, but he should have known. Nicodemus was a scholar of the Torah and God talks about changing the hearts of man and putting his Spirit into the people of Israel in the Old Testament. Here are two examples found in Deuteronomy and Ezekiel.

Deuteronomy 30:6 NLT

The Lord will change your heart and the hearts of all your descendants, so that you will love him with all your heart and soul and so you may live!

Ezekiel 36:26-27 NLT

And I will give you a new heart, and I will put a new spirit in you. I will take out your stony, stubborn heart and give you a tender, responsive heart. And I will put my Spirit in you so that you will follow my decrees and be careful to obey my regulations.

John 3:3-6 NLT

Jesus replied, "I tell you the truth, unless you are born again, you cannot see the Kingdom of God." "What do you mean?" exclaimed Nicodemus. "How can an old man go back into his mother's womb and be born again?" Jesus replied, "I assure you, no one can enter the Kingdom of God without being born of water and the Spirit. Humans can reproduce only human life, but the Holy Spirit gives birth to spiritual life. So don't be surprised when I say, "You must be born again."

The first appearance of the Holy Spirit in the New Testament is found when the Holy Spirit visits Mary and produces in her the baby Jesus. (Matthew Chapter 1)

John the Baptist

Luke 1:14-17 NLT

You will have joy and gladness, and many will rejoice at his birth, for he will be great in the sight of the Lord. He must never touch wine or other alcoholic drinks. He will be filled with the Holy Spirit, even before his birth. And he will turn many Israelites to the Lord their God. He will be a man with the spirit and power of Elijah. He will prepare the people for the coming of the Lord.

God instills the Holy Spirit in John the Baptist before he was born. John the Baptist is filled with Holy Spirit. The *spirit* as Elijah would imply that they are the same Spirit in both the Old and New Testament.

Zechariah who is John the Baptist's father is filled with the Holy Spirit. He tells of a prophecy regarding his son and the coming of Jesus. The end of Chapter 1 says that John the Baptist grew and became strong in the Spirit. John the Baptist was in the wilderness until the day he appeared publicly to Israel. John the Baptist baptized with water, but Jesus will baptize with the Holy Spirit. The Holy Spirit descended upon Jesus after he was baptized by John the Baptist.

Simeon

Luke 2:25-32 NLT

At that time there was a man in Jerusalem named Simeon. He was righteous and devout and was eagerly waiting for the Messiah to come and rescue Israel. The Holy Spirit was upon him and had revealed to him that he would not die until he had seen the Lord's Messiah. That day the Spirit led him to the Temple. So when Mary and Joseph came to present the baby Jesus to the Lord as the law required, Simeon was there. He took the child in his arms and praised God, saying, Sovereign Lord, now let your servant die in peace, as you have promised. I have seen your salvation, which you have prepared for all people. He is a light to reveal God to the nations, and he is the glory of your people Israel!"

Through the power of the Holy Spirit, Simeon could see Jesus through a different paradigm or set of eyes—eyes that see as God wanted him to see! Jesus' parents were amazed that Simeon could know this.

Jesus

Luke 3:21-22 NLT

One day when the crowds were being baptized, Jesus himself was baptized. As he was praying, the heavens opened, and the Holy Spirit, in bodily form, descended on him like a dove. And a voice from heaven said, "You are my dearly loved Son, and you bring me great joy."

Luke 4:1-2 NLT

Then Jesus, full of the Holy Spirit, returned from the Jordan river. He was led by the Spirit in the wilderness, where he was tempted by the devil for forty days.

Jesus was filled by the Holy Spirit after His baptism. He then began His ministry.

Luke 4:14-15 NLT

Then Jesus returned to Galilee, filled with the Holy Spirit's power. Reports about him spread quickly through the whole region. He taught regularly in their synagogues and was praised by everyone.

Jesus tells the disciples that He will send the Holy Spirit to them after He ascends to heaven.

Luke 24:49 NLT

"And I will send the Holy Spirit, just as my Father promised. But stay here in the city until the Holy Spirit comes and fills you with power from heaven."

Pentecost

Acts 2:1-6 NLT

On the day of Pentecost, all the believers were meeting together in one place. Suddenly, there was a sound from heaven like the roaring of a mighty windstorm, and it filled the house where they were sitting. Then, what looked like flames or tongues of fire appeared and settled on each of them. And everyone present was filled with the Holy Spirit and began speaking in other languages, as the Holy Spirit gave them this ability. At that time there were devout Jews from every nation living in Jerusalem.

The Holy Spirit or God's Presence on Earth

When they heard the loud noise, everyone came running, and they were bewildered to hear their own language being spoken by the believers.

The Holy Spirit is now available to anyone who believes that Jesus Christ is their Lord and Savior. Jesus told the disciples to stay in Jerusalem until the Holy Spirit comes. Christians need the power of the Holy Spirit to be complete. Jesus knew that they would need the strength of the Holy Spirit to accomplish the tasks that laid before them.

In the Old Testament, you see the Holy Spirit appear in the second verse of Genesis. You don't see the name of Holy Spirit very often in the Old Testament, but you do see the reference to the Holy Spirit by other names: the Spirit of God, Spirit of the Lord, and others. Obviously, He is part of the Triune God and was present in the beginning. He spent time with Adam and Eve, until they sinned. The Holy Spirit appears to have left earth at that time, except for specific instances.

The people of Israel kept rebelling or turning away from God. They didn't have the advantage that you do today, as you can depend on the power of the Holy Spirit in you. But even with that, your sinful nature always tries to take over and cause you to sin against the will of God in your life. God would send the Holy Spirit to the leaders that He chose in the Bible to help his people.

As in the examples that I covered, He gave them power, strength, wisdom, ability to perform miracles, and He provided them guidance. He encouraged them. He told them that He would always be with them. But as soon as the leader passed on, the people of Israel would turn away from God. The Law of Moses was unable to save mankind, because of its weak sinful nature.

In the New Testament, the Holy Spirit returns to earth permanently, as described in Acts. God knows that you and I need help in order to follow him, so He sent his Son as a sacrifice for our sins. God sent His Spirit to dwell inside you as your support structure, for keeping you on the pathway to follow Him. The Holy Spirit transforms you to be more like Jesus. The Holy Spirit, through the connection of your spirit, helps restrain you from sinning. The Holy Spirit give you the fruit of the Spirit, gifts of the Spirit, and strength to live your life following His commands.

The Holy Spirit is the portion of the Triune God that you have a continual relationship with as he is connected to you or is inside of you. God is still in heaven on his throne with Jesus sitting on his right hand side.

The Holy Spirit has been described in the Bible as having a variety of titles, powers, characteristics, and/or attributes.

- In Isaiah Chapter 11, the Spirit of the Lord is described as providing wisdom and understanding, counsel and might, and knowledge and fear of the Lord.
- In John Chapter 16, the Holy Spirit is described as the Advocate, convicts the world of its sin, guide people to truth, tell of the future, and the Holy Spirit will tell you whatever Jesus reveals to the Spirit.
- In John Chapter 14, the Holy Spirit will teach and remind you of what Jesus taught the world.
- In Romans Chapter 8, the Holy Spirit has the power of life-giving which has freed you. The Holy Spirit helps you in your weakness. The Holy Spirit prays to the Heavenly Father for us with groanings that cannot be expressed in words.
- In 1 Corinthians Chapter 2, the Holy Spirit gives you the words to explain spiritual truth.
- In Ephesians Chapter 1, The Holy Spirit is God's guarantee of your inheritance and that He has purchased you to be his. The Greek word translated to Advocate also means Comforter, Counselor, and Encourager.

- The Holy Spirit is the agent of creation, the method God uses to interact with man, empowering, divine authentication of Kings, provides instruction, holiness, peace, Spirit is lifting, encourager, testifies who Jesus is, inspires, and sanctifies.
- The Holy Spirit provides the fruits and gifts of the Spirit.

There are many more; but you can see that life without the Holy Spirit, is not going to be very fulfilling.

The Holy Spirit provided the information and knowledge that the authors of the Bible relied on to write the sixty-six books of the Bible. The Holy Spirit is in the Bible from the beginning to the end.

The Holy Spirit lives inside of Christians. The power of the Holy Spirit helps you journey through this life. As you can see from the descriptions above, the Holy Spirit offers you many things that you can rely on to help you. Letting the Holy Spirit control your mind leads to a life of peace and joy.

As discussed earlier, you receive gifts and bear fruit as the result of the Holy Spirit's connection to you. You have to learn how to listen to your thoughts which can come from the Holy Spirit. In Romans Chapter 8 it says that Christ lives in us because the Spirit gives life. The Spirit of God raised Jesus from the dead and the same Spirit will give immortal life to your mortal body or soul.

I think that one of the most important verses in the Bible that can give you confidence in your relationship with God is found in Romans.

Romans 8:15-17 NLT

Instead, you received God's spirit when he adopted you as his own children. Now we call him, "Abba, Father." For his Spirit joins with our spirit to affirm that we are God's children. And since we are his children, we are his heirs. In fact, together with Christ we are heirs of God's glory.

How fantastic is that! God's Holy Spirit joins with our Spirit.

You are like the mustard seed. The mustard seed is the smallest seed, but it is full of energy waiting to be released. The mustard is dormant, just as our spirits are dormant or held in check inside your body. Your spirit is searching for fulfillment, but cannot flourish on its own. No matter what culture or isolated tribe in Indonesia, man is searching for a creator. Your spirit is yearning for a connection that completes you as the human being that you were created to be.

Just like the mustard seed whose internal components are ready to come alive with the application of water. As you pour water over the mustard seed to release its energy to grow into a tree, you are waiting for the Holy Spirit to pour its living water over you and connect with your spirit. Another analogy for how man's spirit is functioning until the Holy Spirit enters him is like a motor that is only running on one cylinder. There might be enough power to turn on the radio or the lights, but the car is not going anywhere. Once the Holy Spirit enters you, it is like all the cylinders of the engine are now running. The car is now ready to enter the race and win!

That is Jesus's promise to you—that he will baptize you with the Holy Spirit.

Mathew 3:11 NLT

I baptize with water those who repent of their sins and turn to God. But someone is coming soon who is greater than I am—so much greater that I'm not worthy even to be his slave and carry his sandals. He will baptize you with the Holy Spirit and with fire.

The great power and wisdom of God is hidden to many, as their paradigms are not receptive to God's Word. Even as Christians, we have trouble understanding everything that God teaches.

Romans 11:33-36 NLT

Oh, how great are God's riches and wisdom and knowledge! How impossible it is for us to understand his decisions and his ways! For who can know the Lord's thoughts? Who knows enough to give him advice? And who has given him so much that he need to pay it back? For everything comes from him and exists by his power and is intended for his glory. All glory to him forever! Amen.

Joel 2:28 NLT

Then, after doing all those things, I will pour out my Spirit upon all people. Your sons and daughters will prophecy. Your old men will dream and your young men will see visions. In those days I will pour out my Spirit even on servants—men and women.

God's promise that the Holy Spirit would be available to everyone is revealed back in the book of Joel in the Old Testament.

Deuteronomy 29:29 NLT

The Lord our God has secrets known to no one. We are not accountable for them, but we and our children are accountable forever for all that he has revealed to us, so that we may obey all the terms of these instructions.

In 1 Corinthians 2:7 Paul speaks of the wisdom of the mysteries of God that all of the former rulers of the world did not understand. But God's plan was formed before the world was formed. No eye has seen, no ear has heard, and no mind has imagined what God has prepared for those who love Him. God reveals His plan for you through His Holy Spirit. The Holy Spirit reveals God's thoughts and plans, and the other wonderful things that God wants for you. The Holy Spirit is your Skype connection to God.

The Holy Spirit is only available to us because of Jesus' baptism of suffering on the cross. The Holy Spirit is sacred.

Luke 12:10 NLT

Anyone who speaks against the Son of Man can be forgiven, but anyone who blasphemes the Holy Spirit will not be forgiven. If you deny the presence of the Holy Spirit in your life, you will not be forgiven.

The Holy Spirit through your faith that Jesus Christ is your Lord and Savior is the only way to be connected to God, understand God's plans for you, and to receive a pardon for your sins.

1 Corinthians Chapter 2:10 NLT

But it was to us that God revealed these things by his Spirit. For his Spirit searches out everything and shows us God's deep secrets.

In Galatians 5 you find the passage about the Spirit producing fruit in the lives of Christians. Let's take a look at the whole section of Galatians entitled *Living by the Spirit's Power*.

Galatians 5:16-25 NLT

So I say, let the Holy Spirit guide your lives. Then you won't be doing what your sinful nature craves. The sinful nature wants to do evil, which is just the opposite of what the Spirit wants. And the Spirit gives us desires that are opposite of what the sinful nature desires. These two forces are constantly fighting each other, so you are not free to carry out your good intentions. But when you are directed by the Spirit, you are not under obligation to the law of Moses.

When you follow the desires of your sinful nature, the results are very clear: sexual immorality, impurity, lustful pleasures, idolatry, sorcery, hostility, quarreling, jealousy, outbursts of anger, selfish ambition, dissension, division, envy, drunkenness, wild parties, and other sins like these. Let me tell you again, as I have before, that anyone living that sort of life will not inherit the Kingdom of God.

But the Holy Spirit produces this kind of fruit in our lives: love, joy, peace, patience, kindness, goodness, faithfulness, gentleness, and self-control. There is no law against these things! Those who belong to Christ Jesus have nailed the passions and desires of their sinful nature to his cross and crucified them there. Since we are living by the Spirit, let us follow the Spirit's leading in every part of our lives.

These Bible verses are life in a nutshell. Human existence is summarized in these verses. Every day you have to decide between right and wrong. You make decisions that are good or bad. You can choose to eat a second piece of coconut cream pie, even though you know it is bad for you. God has given mankind the power of free will. You can choose to listen to the Holy Spirit or you can choose to ignore the Holy Spirit.

Unfortunately, for way too many people, they choose to please their self-interests, desires, thoughts, and the flesh that rules their lives. Everyone deals with the struggle between your sinful nature and living according to the direction of the Holy Spirit. As you have read previously, living by the Holy Spirit has many benefits spiritually, mentally, and physically.

What would this world look like if people were led by the Holy Spirit? What if the world followed just the two commandments that Jesus gave us? You are to *love the Lord your God with all your heart and with all your soul and with all your strength and with all your mind; and love your neighbor as yourself.* Two simple laws are all that is needed to live according to the will of God. But, very few people are able to accomplish them. Boy, does this world need a revival!

Let the Holy Spirit give you peace, joy, and love.

The Holy Spirit wants to fill your mind, soul, heart and connect with your spirit!

Chapter 9
Tripartite Man
Spirit, Soul, and Body

1 Thessalonians 5:23 NIV
May God himself, the God of peace, sanctify you through and through.
May your whole spirit, soul, and body be kept blameless
at the coming of our Lord Jesus Christ.

In a very small way, man is similar to God. Man is classically described as being made up of three parts or *tripartite*. Obviously, your parts or composition are different from God's, but there are some similarities. You are made in God's image. You do have a spirit and soul, just as God is a spirit with a soul.

There is actually a fourth part that is mentioned over 550 times in the Bible, referred to as your heart. This heart is not the muscle in your chest that pumps blood throughout your body. As an ophthalmologist, I have a very biased point of view. God developed your blood pumping heart, so that it could pump blood to your eyes; so that you could see, perceive, and interact with this marvelous, beautiful, and astounding world that He created for you to live while on earth. The feeling heart is located in the brain, not the chest.

There is a fifth element related to who you are and that is the mind. The mind is mentioned in the Bible 122 times. Later in the chapter, I will discuss what the Bible says about your emotional heart and your mind. The soul and spirit are very closely connected and it may be difficult to distinguish between the soul and spirit. The spirit and soul are so closely connected that only the Word of God can divide them.

Hebrews 4:12 ESV

For the word of God is living and active, sharper than any two-edged sword, piercing to the division of soul and spirit, of joints and marrow, and discerning the thoughts and intentions of the heart.

The question is: What are human beings and what are the characteristics or components that God has instilled into man? Does it make any difference if a person does not know about the difference between the soul, heart, mind, and spirit? Absolutely, it does! Your soul, spirit, mind, and heart are all interwoven together inside of you, but there are some differences. Even though they are subtle differences, there is overlap of the different attributes of man's makeup. You can get a deeper and more meaningful understanding of how to live your life, by knowing more about how you think and understand the world you live in.

How can you as a Christian understand how to live your life or have a God-centered paradigm, if you don't have a good understanding of the difference? How can you grow spiritually as a Christian, if you are not aware of your spirit? Your spirit is your direct connection or conduit to God. How can you manage your soul, heart, and emotions, unless you understand what they are? How can you oversee the interaction of your spirit, soul, heart, and body or flesh? In order to grow spiritually and learn how to let your spirit guide your life, you need to understand the makeup of who you are. Learning about the differences in your spirit and soul will help you grow and mature as a Christian.

I will try to clarify each part of your makeup—spirit, soul, heart, mind, and body. There are a lot of opinions on this subject and I don't profess to understand all the aspects of human beings. The following are my opinions and my best attempt at trying to give you a new understanding of who you are. I will try to define and discuss what the Bible says about His creation and relate it to the medical knowledge that I have in regards to how your mind and body function.

Genesis 2:7 NLT

Then the Lord God formed man from the dust of the ground. He breathed the breath of life into his nostrils, and the man became a living person.

Adam is the Hebrew word for *man*, which also means to be red. Adam was made from the reddish color of clay. I believe that God breathed life into you with your spirit, and I also believe your soul, as well. The original word for the breath of life that God put into us is *chay*. The Aramaic word *chay* means life, sustenance, or alive. The word chay is almost always used as plural in the Bible. Therefore, I believe that the Bible says that God breathed into your nostrils your spirit and soul.

It makes sense that your spirit and soul reside in your brain, as the Bible tells us that God breathed life into our nostrils, which is right in front of your brain. Obviously, the Holy Spirit may be connected to every cell in your body. Since the decision making and consciousness portion of the brain occurs in the prefrontal cortex, and the Holy Spirit's interaction and communication takes place in the brain, it is the most likely the location where your spirit would be active and working.

There are studies that report that people who have seizures involving their right temporal report having religious experiences. So some of the spirit and soul activity also resides in the temporal lobe. All of your brain or mind is tightly woven with your spirit and soul. No one knows for sure exactly where your soul and spirit are located in your brain. I believe the spirit and soul reside in all the cerebral hemispheres and central nervous system. From there it can extend out to all areas of your body. Your soul can decide to let your spirit dominant your behavior or allow your body (flesh) to dominant your actions. Let's dive into who you really are.

The Body

The Greek word for body is *soma*. Our bodies were made by God to serve as a vessel or reservoir for your spirit and soul while you are on earth. Genesis 2:7 states that God breathed life into us and we became a living being. That breath contained your spirit and soul. Our bodies are full of sensory receptors. As I noted in the chapter about our brains, more than fifty percent of brain activity is receiving, processing, internalizing, filtering, and constantly making decisions about the sensory input received from your bod, even if most of those are subconscious. The amygdala and limbic system are always trying to stimulate you into what the Bible calls *sins of the flesh*. You need to have a balance between your spirit, soul, and body.

As a Christian, you need to pay special attention to the directions of your spirit which is connected to the Holy Spirit, in order to keep your bodily impulses under control. You need to take care of your body, as it is the temple of God's Holy Spirit in you. As stated before, the Seventh Day Adventists very much believe in this and make it a central point on how they live their lives. Without your soul and spirit, your body is without life.

Ecclesiastes 12:7 NLT

For then the dust will return to the earth, and the spirit will return to God who gave it.

Psalm 139:13-14 NIV

For you created my inmost being; you knit me together in my mother's womb. I praise you because I am fearfully and wonderfully made; your works are wonderful; I know full well.

1 Corinthians 6:19 NIV

Don't you realize that your body is the temple of the Holy Spirit, who lives in you and was given to you by God.

You are to take care of your body as it is the residence or temple of your spirit and soul. As I discussed in the chapter on health, the Bible instructs us on how to live a healthy life. There are many studies about what you should eat. The best diet plan appears to be a Mediterranean diet. You should be active and do moderate exercise. You need to trust in God to keep the stress and worry out of your life as much as possible. Turn it all over to Him. As I discussed before, fear, anxiety, stress, and anger are the major causes of mental illness and disease in modern societies.

1 John 4:16-18 NLT

We know how much God loves us, and we have put our trust in his love. God is love, and all who live in love live in God and God lives in them. And as we live in God, our love grows more perfect. So we will not be afraid on the day of judgement, but we can face him with confidence because we live like Jesus here in this world. Such love has no fear, because perfect love expels all fear.

The Soul

What is our soul? First, the soul is immortal, if you are a believer in Christ.

Mathew 10:28 NLT

Don't be afraid of those who want to kill your body; they cannot touch your soul. Fear only God, who can destroy both the soul and the body.

Genesis 35:18 NLV

As Rachel's soul was leaving, for she died, she gave him the name Benoni.

There are many points of view as to what is the soul. Over the course of history, many people have written extensively about it. Needless to say, that understanding of what is the soul is complicated. We will never completely understand what it is. In the Bible, many times people are called souls.

Exodus 31:14 KJV

Ye shall keep the Sabbath therefore; for it is holy unto you: every one that defileth it shall surely be put to death: for whosoever doeth any work therein, that soul shall be cut off from among his people.

Proverbs 11:30 NLV

The fruit of those who are right with God is a tree of life, and he who wins souls is wise.

1 Peter 2:25 NLT

Once you were like sheep who wandered away. But now you have turned to your Shepherd, the Guardian of your souls.

Many times in the Bible, God refers to man as a soul. In simplest terms, it is who you are. I am Jim Croley. I have a particular set of emotions, personality, thoughts, desires, loves, attributes, and abilities. Your soul is composed of your intellect, will, emotions, personality, tendencies, dispositions, self-awareness, evaluates, judges, abstract thinking, mental state, relationships, and volition. Your soul is the part of you that worships and praises God.

Psalm 103:1-2 KJV

Bless the Lord, O my soul: and all that is within me, bless his holy name. Bless the Lord, O my soul, and forget not all his benefits:

Luke 1:46 NLT

Mary responded, "Oh, how my soul praises the Lord."

Definition and origin of soul.

In the Old Testament the Hebrew word for soul is *nepes*. It appears in the Old Testament nearly 500 times. In the King James version of the Bible, the word *nepes* is translated into 42 different English words or terms.

The definition of soul is the spiritual or immaterial part of a human being regarded as immortal. In the New Testament, the word for soul is *psuche* which means heart, life, or mind. The word soul appears in the New Testament 55 times. Other definitions for psuche is breath, the soul, vital breath, life, and breath of life. It is the root word for the English word psyche. It is also where we get the term psychology, psychologist, or psychiatrist, which is the study or treatment of the soul or mind.

Psychostasia is from the Greek meaning weighing of souls. It is a method of divine determination of fate, which has persisted from the Iliad on through Christian theology. People have been trying to weigh the soul in the body as far back as ancient Egyptian times. In Egyptian mythology, Duat is the underworld; this is where the weighing of the heart would take place. This was judged by Anubis using a feather representing Ma'at. Ma'at is the goddess of truth and justice. The heart was at the center of life – spirit Ka. There is an Egyptian tomb painting from 2,500 BC depicting the soul being weighed.

The most quoted reference to the weight of the soul occurred on March 10, 1907 in the New York Times. It reported on an experiment by Dr. Duncan Macdougall. He placed six patients dying from tuberculosis on a large platform scale. He measured the difference in their body weight immediately before and after death. He concluded that the soul weighed twenty-one grams. There were problems with the procedures and interpretations of the results, but this is the most reported weight of the soul.

Noetic Science performed experiments on a large number of people. They found that the soul weighed 1/3000th of an ounce. Similar experiments were performed on two hundred people and reported the same weight loss—1/3000th of an ounce. In 1990, Lyall Watson found in his experiments that the body weight decreased by 2.5 to 6.0 grams at death. Eugenyus Kugis in 2006 at the Institute of Semiconductor of

Lithuania Academy of Science, found that the weight loss at death was between 3 to 7 grams.

Using Dark Plasma Theory, scientists measured the weight of the soul at 10^8. There have been different scientists who have tried to X-Ray or image the soul as it leaves the body.

All these experiments are interesting to learn about, contemplate, and discuss. I don't think we know if the soul and spirit have mass and/or weight. Maybe the spirit and soul are lighter than air, like helium. It is possible that we should weigh more and not less after we die. God did breathe life into Adam and we don't know its composition. If people are waiting to believe in God, because we can weigh the soul; they are putting their beliefs on quicksand, not solid ground. As I discussed earlier, the people of Israel saw first-hand the power and presence of God and they still turned away from Him. The Jewish people crucified Christ who is God. The soul may or may not have weight, but each of us have a soul. It is who you are.

The soul is the connection between your spirit and your body. The soul receives information from the spirit, which in Christians is connected to the Holy Spirit and is your conduit to God. The soul chooses what information it wants to use and makes the decisions that direct your life. The soul is the judge, decision maker, or regulator of all the information your brain is receiving. Your soul is in charge. It controls the amount of influence that your spirit and body have in your life. The soul is the center of your will. When you hear that small voice or a thought that pops up in your mind, it is your spirit and the Holy Spirit communicating with you. It could also be bad thoughts coming from your limbic system or flesh influenced by Satan or his followers.

Creating a God-centered paradigm improves and refines the connection between your spirit and the Holy Spirit. This communication is where your conscience helps direct your life. God instilled that conscience into man. You instinctually know the difference between right and wrong. Your will is found in your soul. Your will is the crucial part of who you are and determines the decisions you make in your life. You will make better decisions, if your soul is closely connected to the influence of the Holy Spirit.

Adam and Eve were initially governed by their spirit and soul. They did not know about the sinful side of the body until their fall. Let's examine their lives. These are my thoughts and interpretations.

Adam and Eve are living their lives in paradise. God put Adam in charge of paradise and let him choose the names of all the animals. He was a vegetarian, as he ate fruits and plants. Adam and Eve's amygdala and limbic systems are essentially dormant. They are living souls that are totally in tune with their spirits. God spoke and communicated with them on a regular basis. The sinful nature of their body or flesh was unknown to them. They have never experienced fear, anxiety, stress, or worry.

Once they sinned against God, their amygdala and limbic system were now turned on and being stimulated. They were suddenly filled with new sensations from their limbic system that they had never experienced. They looked at each other with different eyes or paradigms and felt ashamed. They clothed themselves in order to decrease the stimulation of their new aroused limbic systems. They realized that they had disobeyed God. They knew that they were different. There were new sensations and emotions that they had never experienced. They had become aware of another side of their bodies or flesh.

Adam and Eve tried to hide from God, so that He would not see the transformation in them. Since that time, man has had to battle with the sinful nature of his flesh. The soul struggles to control the limbic system. Can you imagine how Adam and Eve must have felt after they sinned? They went from living in paradise without any cares, worries, or concerns—to suddenly being overwhelmed with new emotions, fears, anxiety, and worries. We still continue dealing with those same problems today.

If your soul allows your spirit to be guided by the Holy Spirit once you have believed in Jesus Christ, then you will live a life that is centered on God. If a man's soul willfully decides to obey God, it will allow man's spirit to control his actions and thoughts. If the soul decides to follow the impulses of your amygdala and limbic system or what the Bible refers to as the flesh, you will not follow God's teachings or direction.

As I discussed earlier, this lifestyle of over stimulating your limbic system leads to medical problems or diseases, poor mental health, and shortened life span. Obviously, there are exceptions to this, as many people can live a long healthy life without being a Christian. But, living a God-centered life greatly increases your chance of living a long, joy filled, and happy life.

As I have said many times, your brain is constantly processing information from your body's senses. Over fifty percent of brain activity is used to simulate and manage the information from your body. The soul is the center of your entire being. The soul decides to let the secular world rule your life or let the spiritual world dominate your thoughts. The soul is the center of your will. The soul makes the decisions in your life. Many people feel that the soul is the center or core of your passions, desires, hate, lusts, and love.

I think that our amygdala and limbic systems are the sources of much of those feelings. The limbic system is the source of your lusts, desires, passions, and what the Bible refers to as your flesh. The soul can succumb or react to these feelings. The will of your soul can choose to listen to them or through the strength of the Holy Spirit control the feelings.

The soul will always tend to listen to the flesh of the body. Man's nature is to listen to the desires of his flesh. It is easy to see why, when all that sensory input is coming into the brain. There is a constant battle going on between the spirit and flesh inside of you. The soul needs to be humble, so that the spirit can manage or rule or have the dominant role in your life. Man will always need help with our souls, which we get from our relationship with God through our faith in Jesus Christ and the Holy Spirit. Here are some Bible verses about your soul.

Psalm 23:3 NIV

He refreshes my soul.

Matthew 11:29 NLT

Take my yoke upon you. Let me teach you, because I am humble and gentle at heart, and you will find rest for your souls.

Psalm 42:1-2 NIV

As the deer pants for streams of water, so my soul pants for you, my God. My soul thirsts for God, for the living God. When can I go and meet with God?

Mathew 22:37 NIV

Jesus replied: Love the Lord your God with all your heart and with all your soul and with all your mind.

Mark 8:36 NIV

What good is it for someone to gain the whole world, yet forfeit their soul?

It is through developing a God-centered paradigm that your soul can develop a strong connection with the Holy Spirit. Your soul will be strengthened, maintained, and provided with rest through your spirit and the Holy Spirit.

The Spirit

The Bible is a spiritual book that tells us about God's love for us, provides us information about God, and gives us instruction on living our lives. In the Old Testament, the Hebrew word for spirit is *ruah*. The word appears in the Old Testament nearly 200 times. Its basic meaning is breath, wind, symbol of life, wind of heaven, source of life, and spirit.

In the New Testament, the Greek word for spirit is *pneuma*. The word appears in the New Testament nearly 400 times. Its basic meaning is the Holy Spirit or the third person of the triune God. It is the spiritual substance by which the human body is made a living person—the essence of an immaterial spirit possessing the power of knowledge, thought, reasoning, and your other mental capacities. It is the life giving spirit. It is your connection or conduit to the Holy Spirit.

Your spirit allows you to pray and have conversations with God. Your spirit helps provide you with the ability to think, contemplate, plan, gives you your intelligence, ability to conceptualize, know right from wrong, and attitude. You have the ability to communicate with other people and put into words your thoughts. The spirit makes your mind different from all other of God's creations, in that you have a mind based on the mind of Christ. When God put your spirit into you, it gave you dominion over all the other creatures on earth.

Job 32:8 NIV

But it is the spirit in a person, the breath of the Almighty, that gives them understanding.

It is the Holy Spirit and your spirit that can give you a different way of thinking or understanding. This is the key to developing a God-centered paradigm. Nurturing and developing a stronger spirit connected to God makes the changes in the brain I previously discussed. Your spirit is extremely important to God, because He wants to fill you with His spirit. The connection to His spirit is your spirit. God is spirit and is similar to the spirit inside of you. You are made in God's image.

Obviously, there are major differences in your spirit and that of God. The first difference is that his Spirit is holy. His Spirit is infinite and pure. His power and knowledge is beyond our ability to understand. He is morally and ethically beyond reproach. He is all knowing and omnipotent. He is the creator of us and the universe. Since God is spirit, He communicates to you through your spirit. He does not live in the physical realm of this world. He communicates with you through the Holy Spirit to the spirit that He placed in you.

You have a spirit that is able to communicate with other spirits. Satan is a spirit and he can influence you in many ways. He can tempt you to sin through stimulating your flesh and mind. He can do it very subtly. Satan is the great deceiver. Everyone needs to improve their perception so that they can recognize him.

The spirit is immortal and returns to God when our physical bodies die. As stated earlier, God breathed into you, your spirit. Your spirit allows you to connect to God through the Holy Spirit. By your connection to the Holy Spirit, your paradigm changes. You can see things that were hidden from your perceptions previously. This is revealed in 1 Corinthians.

1 Corinthians 2:7-16 NLT

No, the wisdom we speak of is the mystery of God—his plan that was previously hidden, even though he made it for our ultimate glory before the world began. But the rulers of this world have not understood it; if they had, they would not have crucified our glorious Lord. That is what the Scriptures mean when they say.

No eye has seen, no ear has heard, and no mind has imagined what God has prepared for those who love him.

But it was to us that God revealed these things by his Spirit. For his Spirit searches out everything and shows us God's deep secrets.

No one can know a person's thoughts except that person's own spirit, and no one can know God's thoughts except God's own Spirit. And we have received God's Spirit (not the world's spirit), so we can know the wonderful things God has freely given us. When we tell you these things, we do not use words that come from human wisdom. Instead, we speak words given to us by the Spirit, using the Spirit's words to explain spiritual truths. But people who aren't spiritual can't receive these truths from God's Spirit. It all sounds foolish to them and they can't understand it, for only those who are

spiritual can understand what the Spirit means. Those who are spiritual can evaluate all things, but they themselves cannot be evaluated by others
For, "Who can know the Lord's thoughts?
Who knows enough to teach him?"
But we understand these things, for we have the mind of Christ.

You can see how important your spirit is, to how you perceive this world and then live your life accordingly. Your spirit is able to perceive and understand things that your soul cannot see or understand. Having a God-centered paradigm is dependent on you using your spirit to perceive and connect with God's Holy Spirit in you. When Adam and Eve sinned, the Holy Spirit was no longer permanently present on earth. The spirit inside man became dormant, or only minimally active. The ability for man to communicate with God was gone, as the Holy Spirit is your connection to God. Man became spiritually dead. The world and society that we have created without the presence and influence of the Holy Spirit is in very sad condition today.

Ephesians 2:1-5 NLT

Once you were dead because of your disobedience and your many sins. You used to live in sin, just like the rest of the world, obeying the devil—the commander of the powers in the unseen world. He is the spirit at work in the hearts of those who refuse to obey God. All of us used to live that way, following the passionate desires and inclinations of our sinful nature. By our very nature we were subject to God's anger, just like everyone else. But God is so rich in mercy, and he loved us so much, that even though we were dead because of our sins, he gave us life when he raised Christ from the dead. (It is only by God's grace that you have been saved!)

Colossians 2:13 NLT

You were dead because of your sins and because your sinful nature was not cut away. Then God made you alive in Christ, for he forgave all your sins.

Your spirit is waiting to be awakened by your acceptance of Jesus Christ as your Savior and receive the Holy Spirit. Once the Holy Spirit enters you, your spirit is released or opened up.

Just like the parable of the mustard seed in Mark 4:30-32, the seed is planted and covered with water, which you read about in the last chapter. The little mustard seed grows to the largest plant in the garden. Your spirit is sitting inside of you yearning to be connected to the Holy Spirit. It's that yearning that many people refer to, when they talk about a hole in your heart that is God shaped. It can only be filled and your heart made whole by God.

People in the most isolated places in the world have a belief in a higher being. They have all kinds of superstitions and beliefs about spirits. Their spirit is desiring a relationship with God. They just have not been exposed to the true God. Many times when these cultures are told about Jesus, large numbers of people are brought to Christ. Their spirit is just waiting for the life-giving water of Jesus Christ.

Your spirit, until it has received the living water is like the mustard seed, it is small and dormant. Similar to the mustard ssed, it is full of nutritional substance for your soul. It just needs the living water from Jesus Christ to release it. The Spirit, being from God, begins to mold you, prune you, and make you a new person. Once you accept Jesus Christ as your Savior, you are transformed or become a new creature. The combining of the Holy Spirit with your spirit turns you into a different person. The most phantasmagorical paradigm shift of all time has occurred!

2 Corinthians 5:17 NLT

Therefore, if anyone is in Christ, the new creation has come; the old has gone, the new is here!

Romans 12:2 NLT

Do not conform to the pattern of this world, but be transformed by the renewing of your mind.

The Greek word for transform is *metamorphoo* which means a total change from the inside out. It is a compound word comprised of *meta* which means change and *morphe* which means form. Form means having a special or certain characteristic form or feature of a person or thing. The English word metamorphosis comes from this word.

There are two kinds of metamorphosis: incomplete and complete. Incomplete indicates that there are changes, but you can still recognize the object or animal from its previous state. Complete metamorphosis is that you cannot recognize the new animal from its previous self. There is no resemblance at all—such as in the case of caterpillar and a butterfly. They have the same DNA or genomic equivalence, but they look completely different.

A butterfly lays these very small eggs. These eggs hatch into a caterpillar. The caterpillar grows rapidly and when fully developed changes to the pupa stage. This is known as the chrysalis. This is the most astonishing stage in the process of metamorphosis. The outer skin of the caterpillar becomes the chrysalis or shell. The caterpillar inside this shell dissolves into a total liquid state. Nothing of the caterpillar visibly remains. It is now just a glop of amorphous liquid. It is through the process of metamorphosis, that it emerges as a beautiful butterfly. Even though the same DNA is present, the butterfly is completely and totally different from the caterpillar.

You are to mimic that type of metamorphosis from the inside out when you become a Christian and are born again! The spirit inside of you is now made whole by the Holy Spirit. You are a new creature which looks, acts, behaves, and lives differently. As you grow in your relationship with God and Jesus Christ through the Holy Spirit, you continually change. You go through a metamorphosis by becoming more like God. You can never obtain it, but you are to strive towards the goal of righteousness.

Galatians 2:20 NLT

My old self has been crucified with Christ. It is no longer I who live, but Christ lives in me. So I live in this earthly body by trusting in the Son of God, who loved me and gave himself for me.

2 Corinthians 3:17-18 NLT

For the Lord is the Spirit, and wherever the Spirit of the Lord is, there is freedom. So all of us who have had that veil removed can see and reflect the glory of the Lord. And the Lord – who is the Spirit – makes us more and more like him as we are changed into his glorious image.

You are also told to renew your mind and/or soul. Renew comes from the Greek word *anakainoo*. This means to make qualitatively new or move to one stage higher. The Bible says that you are to renew yourself daily.

John 4:23-24 NLT

But the time is coming—indeed it's here now—when true worshipers will worship the Father in spirit and in truth. The Father is looking for those who will worship him that way. For God is Spirit, so those who worship him must worship in spirit and in truth.

The spirit and flesh in man are juxtaposed to each other. Your spirit is trying to influence your soul, just as your flesh is sending signals of its desires. Satan knows that the key to keeping you away from God is through your amygdala and limbic system. Look at all the things the secular world exposes everyone to on TV, radio, social media, and other sources. Your mind is continually being bombarded with horrible and sinful things. Your mind and paradigm are being influenced and changed by this input. This is especially true for children and their young developing brains.

If your emotions, stress, anxiety, fears, anger, and desires are out of control, he wins. You need to strive to humble yourself and let the Holy Spirit be the center of your life. As you do this, your spirit will strengthen with the guidance of the Holy Spirit. Your paradigm will begin to shift to a paradigm that is centered on God.

You have heard of the term about computers, which is, garbage in garbage out. The same goes for diet and food. If you eat food full of calories and lots of it, you are going to be obese and unhealthy. Also the same goes for your mind, heart, spirit, and soul. If you spend more and more of your time and thoughts on God, Jesus, and your connection to the Holy Spirit, you begin to shift your paradigm on God and your spiritual life. Your spirit will begin to govern your soul, as you get closer to God. Then you will begin to experience all the benefits of a God-centered paradigm.

Romans 8:3-4 NLT

The law of Moses was unable to save us because of the weakness of our sinful nature. So God did what the law could not do. He sent his own Son in a body like the bodies we sinners have. And in that body God declared an end to sin's control over us by giving his Son as a sacrifice for our sins. He did this so that the just requirement of the law would be fully satisfied for us, who no longer follow our sinful nature but instead follow the Spirit.

Hebrews 12:9 NLT

Moreover, we have all had human fathers who disciplined us and we respected them for it. How much more should we submit to the Father of Spirits and live!

The key to a God-centered paradigm is listening to the Holy Spirit through your spirit. Your spirit is guided by God through his Holy Spirit. Your soul needs to be guided by your spirit. The spirit needs to be nourished and strengthened on a daily basis. Later in the book, I will go over how you can nourish your spirit and soul resulting in a paradigm shift toward God.

There are several words in the Bible that are translated into spirit, soul, mind, and heart. These words overlap and are used in different contexts. There are two other commons words that are used in the Bible that refer to the characteristics of human beings. These words or terms are mind and heart. What do these terms mean in terms of who you are?

Ezekiel 14:5 NLT

I will do this to capture the minds and hearts of all my people who have turned from me to worship their detestable idols.

Hebrews 10:16 NLT

Says the Lord: I will put my laws in their hearts, and I will write them on their minds.

I think that these verses are a reference to the two components of the soul which are the mind and heart. Since your soul is who you are as a person, then the soul thinks and has feelings.

Mind

Earlier in this chapter, I quoted Bible verses from 1 Corinthians. Verse 16 says that we have the mind of Christ. God has given man the ability to think. As I said, I believe that the mind in the Bible is the thinking portion of your soul. We think of our brains and minds interchangeably. Our brains create our thoughts.

The Hebrew word most commonly related to your mind in the Old Testament is *leb* or *lebab*. This means inner man, mind, will, and heart. The Greek word most commonly used in the New Testament is *nous*. This means mind, understanding, reason, the reasoning faculty, intellect, knowledge, and reflective thinking. For Christians, it is the God-given ability to think. Another Greek term used in the Bible for mind is *dianoia*. This means critical thinking or thorough reasoning.

It is in your mind that willful decisions are made. These decisions are made in your prefrontal cortex. The Bible states that your mind is where you make decisions, judgments, and is the location of your will or volition. As I stated before, your mind is very busy. Over fifty percent of your brain is used to receive and process sensory input from your body.

You may have as many as 75,000 thoughts pass through your mind a day. It can be very easy to get caught up in all those thoughts, desires, and ideas.

Satan is delighted to use this large volume of information to his advantage, so that you don't focus your life on God. He wants to keep people's brains busy and confused especially their limbic systems. Satan's goal is to keep your amygdala revved up so that you lose focus. Satan can be very subtle. He doesn't have to always entice you with sinful thoughts or desires to get what he wants. He just has to keep your mind busy with secular things in this world, so that your mind does not have time to think about God.

People are always saying that they are too busy when they need an excuse not to do something. Man's priority needs to be God first, everything else is second.

Colossians 3:2 NLT

Set your minds on things above, not on earthly things.

In Ephesians chapter 4 we are told to put off your old self or former behavior and be renewed in the spirit of your mind. You are to have a new attitude in your mind and change how you think. You are called to be more Christ-like.

Romans 8:5-6 NLT

Those who are dominated by the sinful nature think about sinful things, but those who are controlled by the Holy Spirit think about things that please the Spirit. So letting your sinful nature control your mind leads to death. But letting the Spirit control your mind leads to life and peace.

Here are three Bible verses from Mathew 22:37, Mark 12:30, and Luke 10:27 that tell us how to love God which are the same.

*You must love the Lord your God
with all you heart, all your soul, and all your mind.*

Heart

When you think, plan, contemplate, or reason, you are using your mind. When you feel happiness, sadness, pleasure, fear, or anger, you are reacting to your emotional responses in your limbic system. The heart is the emotional portion of your soul. When the Bible references the heart, it is not talking about the muscle in your chest that pumps blood. It is talking about the emotional and feeling part of your soul. People commonly use the word *heart* when they talk about their emotions. The word *heart* occurs almost one thousand times in the Bible.

In the Old Testament, the word for heart is the Hebrew word *lebab*—which is used for heart and is interchangeable with mind. It means the inner most organ, courage, mind, and midst. In the New Testament, the Greek word for heart is *kardia*. You may recognize this word, which is used for medical terms for the heart or cardiac. It means the middle, feelings, inner self, core, or where a person believes and has faith. So, the feeling or emotional heart is located in the brain.

Other words that are translated as heart are *ranz* (reins) and *nephros* (kidneys). *Ranz* means heart, inward parts, kidneys, or reins. Hebrew psychology recognizes reins as the location of the deepest emotions or affections of man, which only God can fully know. The Hebrew word for kidneys is *kilyah* which is translated as the seat of emotions. The Greek word is *nephros* which means the inner most portion of the mind. You may recognize the word *nephros* which is the origin of the specialty in medicine called nephrology.

God has a heart as well.

Acts 13:22 NLT

God said, I have found David son of Jesse, a man after my own heart.

Jeremiah 3:15 NLT

And I will give you shepherds after my own heart, who will guide you with knowledge and understanding.

The heart feels negative emotions such as sorrow, bitterness, fear, anger, anxiety, pride, envy, and other negative emotions. The heart feels positive emotions such as happiness, gladness, joy, peace, passion, cheerfulness and, most importantly, love. You are to love God with all your heart. The heart needs to be renewed and regenerated constantly. Your soul's emotions, feelings, or heart needs to be controlled by your spirit connected to God. Sin is first committed in the heart.

Mark 7:21-23 NLT

For from within, out of a person's heart, come evil thoughts, sexual immorality, theft, murder, adultery, greed, wickedness, deceit, lustful desires, envy, slander, pride, and foolishness. All these vile things come from within; they are what defile you.

Jeremiah 17:9-10 NLT

The human heart is the most deceitful of all things, and desperately wicked. Who really knows how bad it is? But, I the Lord, search all hearts and examine secret motives. I give all people their due rewards, according to what their actions deserve.

Your heart or emotion is the starting point where sin is generated. Your limbic system is the part of the brain where this occurs. God knows about all your inner thoughts and desires.

As discussed in the chapter on the health benefits of a God-centered paradigm, a joyful, happy, and peaceful heart leads to a longer life. This is noted in Proverbs.

Proverbs 17:22 NLT

A cheerful heart is good medicine, but a broken spirit saps a person's strength.

In the three bible verses about loving God with all your heart, soul, and strength, the heart is always mentioned first. You are to love God with your inner most being or core.

When we think of the words reins and kidneys in regards to your heart or emotions, you can get a little different perspective on your inner self. Reins are used to control horses. You use reins to control, guide, and direct the horse so that you make it to your destination.

Your soul determines who you are and what you want to accomplish in life. Kidneys have a different function in your body. The kidneys filter out the impurities in your body. As the blood passes through the kidneys, it filters out the impurities in your blood.

Your soul needs to control your brain and remove impurities from your life. The priority of the soul is to follow the guidance of the Holy Spirit. The Holy Spirit, through your soul, is to guide your life like using reins. The Spirit is to also help you stay away from sin or impurities, as the kidneys keep your body clean from bad chemical or elements in your body.

The tripartite man and woman need to grow and mature in their relationship with God. Your body need to be cared for, as it is the temple of the Holy Spirit. Also your soul and mind needs to be continually renewed as it says in Romans 12:2.

An interesting analogy is the eagle. As the eagle matures, it goes through a molting process. The juvenile eagle begins to lose its secondary down and grow feathers. The feathers of the juvenile eagle are thicker and longer than an adult eagle. This makes the juvenile eagle's flight clumsy and slow. As the eagle becomes an adult, the molting process continues. The feathers become more streamlined and shorter. This increases the speed and grace by which the eagle can fly. Even as adults, they are slowly molting or growing new feathers. The old feathers become worn and tattered. The eagle needs to be continually renewed in order to maintain its speed and agility.

So, it is with humans. We need to continually clean out the bad things in our lives and replace them with fruits of the Holy Spirit.

Isaiah 40:31 NLT

But those who trust in the Lord will find new strength. They will soar high on wings like eagles. They will run and not grow weary. They will walk and not faint.

This is similar to the growth of Christians as they mature in their faith. You need to shed or change your paradigm toward a closer relationship with God. To live a God-centered paradigm or life, you need to be constantly working and striving to keep your focus on God. You are not to be conformed to this world, but transformed by renewing your mind on God on a daily basis.

Toward the end of the book, I will discuss ways and techniques to help stabilize and improve how the brain functions.

The Lord calls you to love Him totally and completely.

You are to love Him with purpose and passion!

Chapter 10
How Much God Loves You

John 3:16 NLT
For this is how God loves the world:
He gave his one and only Son,
so that everyone who believes in him
will not perish but have eternal life.

The above verse is a very obvious place to start, when talking about God's love for you. That Jesus came to earth to die for your and my sins, because He loved us, is an historical fact. It is recorded by Flavius Josephus, who was a Jewish historian. He recorded this in his writings called *The Antiquities of the Jews*. This is not an apologetics book, but I think it is good to start from a factual basis. Jesus was on earth and was crucified by Pontius Pilate. He rose again on the third day and was seen by many of His followers. On the surface, you might think that it's really nice that He cares or loves you.

The word *love* is probably the most misused word in the English language. We love everything and everyone. We love ice cream, football, food, watching TV, truffles, vacation, skiing, sailing, and on and on and on! Love has been so over used that for many, it has lost its true meaning.

Let's take a little deeper look into God's love. Since the very beginning, man has failed to live up to God's expectations. Adam and Eve failed to follow one simple rule that God had given them. The chosen people of Israel have been a problem from day one. They ignored His laws and repeatedly turned away from Him. They worshipped others gods or idols. God sent the Messiah to save them and they killed Him. Today, the Jewish people still don't recognize Jesus as God's Son.

We are like the black sheep in the family, as we fail to keep our focus on God. Yet, He still loves each and every one of us. You are His creation and His love for you has never wavered. The Bible is God's love letter to you. It tells you of His love, instructs you about your physical health, mental health, diet, instructs you on daily living, and to love one another. Let's go back over the different types of love found in the Bible.

There are four Greek words used for love in the Bible. The word *Phileo* is the word for love between friends, which means affection, fondness, or liking. This is where the city of Philadelphia gets its name, the city of brotherly love. This type of love involves giving as well as receiving. It may or may not be permanent; and it can end under distress.

The word *Eros* for love is erotic love. It is the love of passion. It is based on emotions in the body. This love also can be temporary depending on the person's emotions, which can wax and wane.

The word *Storge* for love is natural affection. It is the love for family, husband, wife, or child.

The word *Agape* for love is based on the preciousness of the subject loved, as it is unconditional love. It is not based on worth, feelings, emotions, or merit. This love continues to love even when the loved one is unworthy, does not return the love, is not lovable, is mean or unresponsive. It desires only good for the other. It originates from God's nature. God loves you with agape love. You don't deserve it. God loves you anyway and unconditionally. You don't even have to ask for it, as God loved you first. It is the purist or most perfect word for love in the Greek language. God is love.

The parable of the prodigal son is one of my favorites. It is found in Luke Chapter 15. There have been many commentaries and sermons on the parable. I am going to focus on the father. This is my version of the story. The younger son goes to his father and asks for his inheritance. The father agrees to give him his inheritance. The son goes away and wastes all his money on all kinds of sinful things. There was a famine at the time and the son began to starve. He worked for a local farmer feeding his pigs. His starvation got to the point that even the slop he was feeding the pigs began to look tasty. He finally decided that he had no choice; he would return home to face the humiliation and consequences of his actions. He would even be willing to work as one of his father's slaves.

You can imagine him walking back home, with his head lowered from the embarrassment and shame. His clothes are dirty and torn. He smells, as he hasn't had a bath in a long while. His hair is a mess and he looks like a lost person. The father sees him when he was still a long way off in the distance. The father could have been upset, as he had heard what his son was doing with his inheritance. He could have waited until his son reached the house and scolded him for what he had done. He could have watched him finish his walk of shame all the way to the house.

(This is what I think is the great part of the story.) Instead, the father was full of compassion and love. He runs to his son, embraces him, and kisses him. He calls for, not just clean clothes, but the finest robe. He gave him a ring for his finger and new sandals. A feast was held in his honor with the killing of the fatted calf.

God loves us and He is running to each and every one of us. The question is, what are you doing? Are you able to perceive Him in your life? Does your paradigm allow you to perceive the Holy Spirit around you and trying to communicate with you? He is there. Just like you saw in the examples of paradigms in the first chapter, many people fail to see or perceive the Holy Spirit. They don't take the time to understand and nurture the relationship of their spirit to the Holy Spirit. In many churches, this relationship is not talked about very much. But is a completely and totally necessary part of living a Christian life or having a God-centered paradigm. The Holy Spirit is the one who is talking to your soul through your spirit.

When you became a Christian, the Holy Spirit is continually communicating with you. If you have not become a Christian, the Holy Spirit is appealing to you to believe in Jesus Christ as your Lord and Savior. Your paradigm may keep you from perceiving the Holy Spirit communicating with you. God loves everyone and wants to share His love with each of us.

When you accept Jesus, God's love enters you through the Holy Spirit. If you want to deepen your relationship with God and feel His love more completely, then allow the Holy Spirit to love you completely. Don't just allow the Holy Spirit to occupy a portion of you. Give the Holy Spirit permanent residence, right smack dab in the middle of your paradigm! Like the song says by Rudimental, *Feel the Love*.

Romans 1:20-21 NLT

For ever since the world was created, people have seen the earth and sky. Through everything God made, they can clearly see his invisible qualities— his eternal power and divine nature. So they have no excuse for not knowing God.

God's love, power, and omnipotence is beyond our knowledge or understanding. He created everything. If you printed out on paper your DNA sequence, the stack of paper would be taller than the Washington Monument in D.C. He loves and knows everything about you. He even knows the number of hairs on your head. He designed your body and knows every gene or cell. That is how much attention and detail He has put into place for you.

Matthew 10:28-31 NLV

Do not be afraid of them who kill the body. They are not able to kill the soul. But fear Him who is able to destroy both the soul and body in hell. Are not two small birds sold for a very small piece of money? And yet not one of the birds falls to the earth without your Father knowing it. God knows how many hairs you have on your head. So do not be afraid. You are more important than many small birds.

Ephesians 3:14-19 NLT

When I think of all this, I fall to my knees and pray to the Father, the creator of everything in heaven and on earth. I pray that from his glorious, unlimited resources he will empower you with inner strength through his Spirit. Then Christ will make his home in your hearts as you trust in Him. Your roots will grow down into God's love and keep you strong. And may you have the power to understand, as all God's people should, how wide, how high, and how deep his love is. May you experience the love of Christ, though it is too great to understand fully. Then you will be made complete with all the fullness of life and power that comes from God.

God's love is beyond your or my understanding. But, isn't it great to know that His love is larger and more fantastic than your mind can even imagine! You have a little bit of an idea, if you are parent. The love you have for your child is a deep sacrificing love. Yet, God's heart is able to love at a level beyond your imagination. The size or depth of His heart is beyond the size of the universe.

Ephesians 3:19 NLT

May you experience the love of Christ, though it is too great to understand fully. Then you will be made complete with all the fullness of life and power that comes from God.

He is involved in every aspect of your life. He has agape love for each and every one of us individually.

John 15:9 NLV

I have loved you just as My Father has loved Me. Stay in My love.

Isaiah 43:4 NLV

You are of great worth in My Eyes. You are honored and I love you.

Proverbs 8:17 NLT

I love all who love me. Those who search will surely find me.

Jeremiah 29:11 NLT

"For I know the plans I have for you," says the Lord. "They are plans for good and not for disaster, to give you future and a hope."

God created you and has a plan for your life. Because He has a plan for you, He will protect you so that you can fulfill His plan. I have needed His help, love, protection, and guidance all my life. Without that I would not be here today.

Maybe the most well-known of Bible passage concerning God's protection is next.

Psalm 23:1-4 NLT

The Lord is my shepherd; I have all that I need. He lets me rest in green meadows; he leads me beside peaceful streams. He renews my strength. He guides me along right paths, bringing honor to his name. Even when I walk through the darkest valley, I will not be afraid, for you are close behind me. Your rod and your staff protect and comfort me.

There are many other Bibles verses that talk about His guidance and protection for you.

2 Samuel 22:2-4 NLT

The Lord is my rock, my fortress, and my savior; my God is my rock, in whom I find protection. He is my shield, the power that saves me, and my place of safety. He is my refuge, my savior, the one who saves me from violence. I called on the Lord, who is worthy of praise, and he saved me from my enemies.

Isaiah 41:10 NLT

Don't be afraid, for I am with you. Don't be discouraged, for I am your God. I will strengthen you and help you. I will hold you up with my victorious right hand.

Isaiah 54:17 NLT

But in that coming day no weapon turned against you will succeed. You will silence every voice raised up to accuse you. These benefits are enjoyed by the servants of the Lord; their vindication will come from me.

2 Thessalonians 3:3 NLT

But the Lord is faithful; he will strengthen you and guard you from the evil one.

Romans 5:5 NLT

And this hope will not lead to disappointment. For we know how clearly God loves us, because he has given us the Holy Spirit to fill our hearts with his love.

You feel God's love through the Holy Spirit in you. Your spirit is connected to God through the Holy Spirit. The more time you spend in reading the Bible, praying, meditating, and spending quiet time with God, the more you will be able to feel and understand God's love for you. Then you are able to follow the second commandment that Jesus gave, which is to love your neighbor as you love yourself.

1 John 4:7-12 NLT

Dear friends. Let us continue to love one another, for love comes from God. Anyone who loves is a child of God and knows God. But anyone who does not love does not know God, for God is love.

God showed how much he loved us by sending His one and only Son into the world so that we might have eternal life through him.

This is real love—not that you loved God, but that he loved you and sent his Son as a sacrifice to take away your sins. Dear friends, since God loved you that much, you surely ought to love others. No one has ever seen God. But if you love one another, God lives in you, and his love is brought to full expression in you.

These Bible verses tell you what life is about. God loved you first. You are instructed to love God with all your heart, soul, mind, and strength. Then, you are to love your neighbor as you love yourself. If only everyone would follow these two commandments, life in this world would be dramatically changed. That would be the paradigm shift of all time for mankind!

We need to understand and accept that God loves us. He loves you with all your sins, faults, and short-comings. If you can learn this, you can love and forgive yourself. For many people, guilt is a heavy burden that they are carrying. They are unable to forgive themselves and therefore are stuck in the quagmire of guilty feelings. God loves you no matter what you have done. He still loves you. If you have turned over your life to God, then Jesus has taken all your sins onto Himself. He not only has forgiven your and my sins, but God no longer remembers them. You need to turn over everything to God and live a new life.

Isaiah 43:25 NLT

I—yes, I alone—will blot out your sins for my own sake and will never think of them again.

Romans 4:7 NLT

Oh, what joy for those whose disobedience is forgiven, whose sins are put out of sight.

Hebrews 8:12 NLT

And I will forgive their wickedness, and I will never again remember their sins.

If God no longer remembers your sins, you need to do the same. You have to release the guilt that paralyzes you. This goes back to the chapter about the health benefits of a God-centered paradigm. God does not condemn you. Therefore, you need to live and enjoy the fruits of the Spirit. Stop focusing on the negative and the guilt. God doesn't remember those things that are causing the negative feelings.

Let God's love change how you think and your paradigm. You have a new beginning in Christ. You can be like the caterpillar and become a beautiful butterfly. You can depend on God being there for you. Nothing can separate you from God's love.

Isaiah 54:10 NLT

For the mountains may move and the hills disappear, but even then my faithful love for you will remain.

Romans 8:35-39 NLT

Can anything ever separate us from Christ's love? Does it mean he no longer loves us if we have trouble or calamity, or are persecuted, or hungry, or destitute, or in danger, or threatened with death? (As the Scriptures say, 'For your sake we are killed every day; we are being slaughtered like sheep.') No, despite all these things, overwhelming victory is ours through Christ, who loved us. And I am convinced that nothing can ever separate us from God's love. Neither death nor life, neither angels nor demons, neither our fears for today nor our worries about tomorrow—not even the powers of hell can separate us from god's love. No power in the sky above or in the earth below—indeed, nothing in all creation will ever be able to separate us from the love of God that is revealed in Christ Jesus our Lord.

That is absolutely fantastic!! God is in charge. Nothing can separate you from God's love. Satan and the secular world will keep trying to interfere with your relationship with God, but will fail in the end. You have the freedom to live your life knowing that you are in God's hands. God loves you no matter what you have done or what you will do. People who feel guilty need stop, as this is harmful to their mental health. God doesn't even remember their wrong doings or sin once they are Christians. That doesn't mean you have a free ticket to do anything you want, but everyone sins and makes mistakes. God will forgive you, if you sincerely pray and repent of your sin.

Many people believe they are not worthy of God's love—they are too bad or have done too many terrible things. All of us have sinned and do not deserve God's love and forgiveness. You are saved by the grace of God and His love for you. All you have to do is believe and have faith that Jesus Christ is your Lord and Savior. You then can start to enjoy the benefits of belonging to Him.

God wants everyone to live a peaceful and joyful life. Your responsibility is to humble yourself, and realize that you are not in charge or control of your life. You are on God's timeline, not yours. Once you are able to understand this, you can start to change your life. You no longer need to fear, worry, or stress over things that you can't control.

As you read in earlier chapters, fear is a huge problem that many people face in their daily lives. The fear of mistakes, fear of failure, fear of something might happen beyond their control, fear of illness, fear of success (as weird as that sounds), fear you aren't good enough, fear you aren't living up to expectations, and death. God is in charge and loves you with unfailing love.

In 2 Corinthians Chapter 12, it says that when we are weak then God will be strong. As I stated earlier, He has a plan for each and every one of us. You just need to trust that God loves you and only wants good for you.

1 Peter 5:6-7 NLT

So humble yourselves under the mighty power of God, and at the right time he will lift you up in honor. Give all your worries and cares to God, for he cares about you.

Ephesians 2:8-10 NLT

God saved you by his grace when you believed. And you can't take credit for this; it is a gift from God. Salvation is not a reward for the good things we have done, so none of us can boast about it. For we are God's masterpiece. He has created us anew in Christ Jesus, so we can do the good things he planned for us long ago.

In today's world, it's all about me and we are in charge. That is just a false sense of security. The world will ultimately always follow God's plans. Your job is to have faith, to love God, and love one another.

1 John 4:7-8 ESV

Dear friends, let us continue to love one another, for love comes from God. Anyone who loves is a child of God and knows God. But anyone who does not love does not know God, because God is love.

You are the only creation of God's that He has instilled into the ability to love. You will give up your life for others. How many men and women of our armed forces have given up their lives for us? If someone is drowning, a stranger will risk their life trying to save that drowning person. That love that God placed in you is special. That is one of the characteristics that makes you similar to God. You have the ability to love.

God also wants you to be passionate about Him. God wants you to love Him with purpose and passion!

Revelation 3:15 NLT

I know all the things you do, that you are neither hot nor cold. I wish that you were one or the other! But since you are lukewarm, neither hot nor cold, I will spit you out of my mouth!

Because God loves you so much, He will be with you always. He knows everything about you. He knows what you are going to do before you do it. This type of love that God has for you reminds me of Psalm 139 by King David.

Psalm 139:1-18 TLB

O Lord, you have examined my heart and know everything about me. You know when I sit or stand. When far away you know my every thought. You chart the path ahead of me and tell me where to stop and rest. Every moment you know where I am. You know what I am going to say before I even say it. You both precede and follow me and place your hand of blessing on my head.

This is too glorious, too wonderful to believe! I can never be lost to your Spirit! I can never get away from my God! If I go up to heaven, you are there; if I go down to the place of the dead, you are there. If I ride the morning winds to the farthest oceans, even there your hand will guide me, your strength will support me. If I try to hide in the darkness, the night becomes light around me. For even darkness cannot hide from God; to you the night shines as bright as day. Darkness and light are both alike to you.

You made all the delicate, inner parts of my body and knit them together in my mother's womb. Thank you for making me so wonderfully complex! It is amazing to think about. Your workmanship is marvelous—and how well I know it. You were there while I was being formed in utter seclusion! You saw me before I was born and scheduled each day of my life before I began to breathe. Every day was recorded in your book!

How precious it is, Lord, to realize that you are thinking about me constantly! I can't even count how many times a day your thoughts turn toward me. And when I wake in the morning, you are still thinking of me!

There was a story posted on Facebook by Jack Speed that shows how much God loves you and is there for you. I saw a similar story on the TV show *The Yukon Men*, and there are other traditions about boys becoming men.

This is a story about a man who is teaching his son what it means to become a man. The father takes his son into the woods near the end of the day and gives him three instructions that he has to follow. He is required to sit on a stump the whole night. He cannot remove the blindfold that has been placed over his eyes, until he feels the rays of the morning sun on his face. And he cannot cry out for help. Once he survives the night, he is a man.

The son is obviously scarred the whole night. He hears all kinds of noises, the wind blowing, wild animals nearby, and times of complete eerie silence. The son doesn't move from his stump. Finally, after a long horrible night, the sun appears and he removes his blindfold. He looks around; there is his father sitting on a stump right next to him. The father was there watching his son through the whole night. He loves his son and was there to protect him. The son was never alone sitting there on the stump.

The secular world and Satan want you to keep your blindfold on. They don't want you to perceive and know that God is with you. All you need to do, is take off the blindfold of this world and see with the spiritual eyes of a God-centered paradigm. God is faithful. You can have absolute confidence that He loves you, will never leave you, and is always there for you. Learn to see with God-centered eyes or spiritual eyes.

We tend to bring God down to our level of understanding. As humans, we are unable to understand the completeness and vastness of God's love for us. How great it is to know that God loves you so much! He is thinking about you, watching you, and is holding you in His hands! You are never alone in this world. God is always there for you.

> *One who has been touched by grace will no longer look on those who stray as "those evil people" or "those poor people who need our help." Nor must we search for signs of "love worthiness." Grace teaches us that God loves because of who God is, not because of who we are.*
> *— Philip Yancey*
>
> *No matter what storm you face, you need to know that God loves you. He has not abandoned you.*
> *— Franklin Graham*

Though our feelings come and go, God's love for us does not.
— *C.S. Lewis*

God loves each of us as if there were only one of us.
—*Augustine*

The Bible verses that are most commonly used at weddings are found in 1 Corinthians Chapter 13. This is the love chapter of the Bible. I am only going to share the last three verses. Please take the time to read the entire chapter.

1 Corinthians 13:11-13 NLT

When I was a child, I spoke and thought and reasoned as a child. But when I grew up, I put away childish things. Now we see things imperfectly, like puzzling reflections in a mirror, but then we will see everything with perfect clarity. All that I know now is partial and incomplete, but then I will know everything completely, just as God now knows me completely.

Three things will last forever—faith, hope, and love—and the greatest of these is love.

These are Paul's final words to the Corinthians.

2 Corinthians 13:11 NIV

Finally, brothers and sisters, rejoice! Strive for full restoration, encourage one another, be of one mind, live in peace. And the God of love and peace will be with you.

Jesus took on all the sin of mankind, that man has ever or will commit. He knew what the consequences and severity of doing this was going to be. It is beyond our imagination what pain and suffering Jesus would have to endure because of our sins. His pain, anxiety, and stress were so intense, that blood began to pour from his sweat glands on the Mount of Olives on the Thursday before His crucifixion.

In the movie, The Son of God, there is a scene that made the movie for me and showed God's love for me. Many people may not have paid too much attention to it. Jesus had just been through this horrible scourging and He had been flogged nearly to the point of death. He was knocked to the ground and told to take up His cross. As He crawls over to the cross, you can see the intense agony and pain in his face.

The director inserts the next scene (which probably did not happen), but it is a great illustration of God's love for us. Jesus looks into the camera and suddenly His face changes from this painful distorted look to a beautiful smile, and He kisses the cross. Instantly, you see the pain return to His face.

That brief moment touched my heart and soul. To me, that vividly showed the extent of God's love for me. Isn't it unbelievable to think that Jesus loves you that much? That He was willing to be humiliated and tortured for you. He died on the cross, because He loved you and all people. He knew that the cross was necessary for you to enter His Kingdom. Even though He was suffering, He smiled; because this was His gift that He was giving to you and me.

That scene, which lasted only a second or two, made the movie for me. I thought, "How awesome is our Triune God and His love."

God is LOVE!

Chapter 11
God in Our Brain

Romans 11:33-34 TLB

Oh, what a wonderful God we have!
How great are his wisdom and knowledge and riches!
How impossible it is for us to understand his decisions and his methods!
For who among us can know the mind of God?

Neurotheology is the study of religion or religious experiences in neuroscientific terms. It is also known as spiritual neuroscience. It is the study of neural reasons, correlates, or explanations for spiritual experiences, beliefs, or practices. Aldous Huxley first used the term *neurotheology* in his novel, *Island*. There have been and continue to be many scientists who are trying to find a God spot in your brain. Many of these scientists are atheists or nonbelievers in God. They are searching and studying the brain, trying to explain religion on a purely neurological basis. They are trying to prove that religion was created by man. They are trying to make the case that man's brain created God, instead of God creating man and his brain. Their research is focused on showing that the human brain has created God. They believe there is a God spot in the brain.

Our minds are wired for the need of a god. Just like part of the brain is for vision, speech, muscle control, and hearing, there are a group of cells in the brain responsible for you creating a god in your mind. Many of the scientists believe that man created God in his mind, because of the fear of dying. By creating a god, it would relieve the fear. We could depend on him to save us from death. They believe that because of man's fear, man developed neurons in the brain that were able to create a god.

This ability to create a god was passed genetically on through the generations. There is no explanation why that genetic trait was superior and that it was the reason those particular people survived. It was their way of justifying their belief that there is not a real God, just a god that humans needed to create. According to the scientists, the people who were unable to create a god did not survive over time. It doesn't follow any of their Darwin theories. How did fear and creating a god make a person more likely to succeed or be superior to the other people around that person? They could hunt better and were better warriors, if you believe in Darwin's theories. What made them more superior to other people and made them the survivor of the fittest just because they created a god in their minds? Their logic doesn't make a lot of sense to me.

Most people very rarely think about dying, unless they are close to dying from cancer or some other chronic disease—especially when you are young and having children, where you would pass on any genetic information. Young men think that they are superman and invincible. If you try to follow their reasoning, why would you create a god who lays down all these rules? You are having a great time doing anything that you want and you are going to create a god that tells you to stop. Man's nature has always been to do your own thing and not listen to a god. So man decided to create a god on his own to stop his fun because he is afraid, doesn't pass my smell test.

Therefore, according to these scientists, man developed genes to create God. On the road to Damascus when Saul had the encounter with Jesus, was it just that Saul had a hallucination and was blind for three days? Did early Christians lay down their life and their families' lives, suffer persecution, and ridicule for a story they just heard about? Did the several hundred people who saw Jesus after His resurrection also have an hallucination? People who are set on trying to have your brain create God are not looking at the whole picture. Just as the Bible says, they hear and see but do not understand. Their paradigms do not allow them to perceive the God of the universe.

It is true that no matter where you go in the world, even to the most remote places, there is a belief in a higher being. Nearly every culture has built temples and has burial services sending the soul to heaven or dimension. Instead of it being man creating that perception or belief, maybe God instilled into us the need to search or need Him. God placed in us the neural pathways, so that we could recognize Him.

Look at what it says in the last verses of 1 Corinthians Chapter 2.

1 Corinthians 2:11-16 TLB

No one can really know what anyone else is thinking or what he really is like except that person himself. And no one can know God's thoughts except God's own Spirit. And God has given us his Spirit (not the world's spirit) to tell us about the wonderful free gifts of grace and blessing that God has given us. In telling you about these gifts we have even used the very words given to us by the Holy Spirit, not words that we as men might choose. So we use the Holy Spirit's words to explain the Holy Spirit's facts. But the man who isn't a Christian can't understand and can't accept these thoughts from God, which only the Holy Spirit teaches us. They sound foolish to him because only those who have the Holy Spirit within them can understand what the Holy Spirit means. Others just can't take it in. But the spiritual man has insight into everything, and that bothers and baffles the man of the world, who can't understand him at all. How could he? For certainly he has never been one to know the Lord's thoughts, or to discuss them with him, or to move the hands of God by prayer. But, strange as it seems, we Christians actually do have within us a portion of the very thoughts and mind of Christ.

God made our minds to function in a very small way like His. God designed your brain so that He could communicate and reside in it. Christians think with a mind like God. You have many thoughts in your mind that come from God. The people and scientists who are not Christians are never going to understand. Their paradigms will keep them from knowing. They are usually very closed minded and are going to keep searching, until they get the answer they are looking for. They are going to be looking a long time.

We know a lot of information about how the actual cells of the brain work. We still have no idea how the neurons develop thought or our conscience. It is still a mystery. Scientists will keep on trying to reduce God and religion to a particular place in the brain or brain activity. The idea that your brain invented God, or God made your brain so that you would desire a relationship to Him, is like, which was first the chicken or the egg? Did God make you or did you develop from some lower life form?

You have to be very careful about studies and research. If a researcher or company goes into the study with a result already in mind, the results may be very unreliable. Even a good honest researcher needs to be careful, because their own bias or paradigm can consciously or subconsciously affect the results.

I have drug company representatives come to my office all the time. They bring in a study to show that their drug is superior to their competitor's drug. They show me the study documenting the fact. An hour later, the other drug company's representative comes and tells me their drug is superior. They show me their study that shows it is better. They both can't be right. Everyone and every product advertised on TV is the best. No one admits to being second. The problem is that you can develop a study to prove your point. These companies search for one fact in the study where their drug might be superior, but in other parts of the study it may not be as superior. They only show the facts that show their drug to be superior.

Let's look at other research and the history about where God is in the brain.

- Pythagoras around 500 B.C. described the soul with three parts: reason, intelligence, and passion. The soul was located from the heart to the brain. Passion was located in the heart. Reason and intelligence were located in the brain.
- Greek physician Hippocrates in around 400 B.C. thought that the brain was the seat of the mind.
- Claudius Galen was a Roman physician who lived in 129-199 B.C., he dissected the human brain and thought that the soul was in the ventricles, which contains cerebral fluid.
- Leonardo da Vinci thought the soul was located above the optic chiasm behind the nose, where the optic nerves from the eyes meet.
- Lancisi believed that the soul was deep in the middle of the brain in a structure called the corpus callosum.
- Thomas Willis also believed that the soul was located in the middle of the brain, which composed the inner chamber of the soul.
- Albrecht von Haller thought the soul was in the medulla oblongata. This is in the midbrain at the base of the brain. (Ever since I learned that term, I have always liked the sound of it. You can sound pretty smart if you say these two words named for a structure in the midbrain—the medulla oblongata!)
- Wilder Penfield, who lived from 1891 to 1976, is commonly associated with the premise that there is a neurological God spot.

Throughout history, man has tried to locate the soul in the body and find out, where does God come from, in the mind.

Robert Musil said, "We do not have too much intellect and too little soul, but too little intellect in matters of the soul."

Francis Dyson said, "To summarize the situation, we have three mysteries that we do not understand: the unpredictable movements of atoms, the existence of our consciousness, and the friendliness of the universe to life and mind. I am only saying that the three mysteries are probably connected. I do not claim to understand any of them."

Since many people think that God is merely a product created by our minds, maybe we can stimulate the God part of the brain and create God anytime we want. In the 1980s, the God Helmet was invented by Stanley Koren and neuroscientist Michael Persinger to study religious experiences by stimulation of the temporal lobes. The apparatus was placed on the head of a person and produced a weak magnetic field in the area of the temporal lobes. The God Helmet stimulated the brain by transcranial magnetic stimulation. People reported religious experiences during the stimulation. They believed that the temporal lobe was the center of our religious experiences.

A Swedish researcher published a study in December of 2004 stating that the results of the previous study could not be reproduced. The helmet did not produce a god or cause the development of any religious experience. Again, you have to be very careful about what a study says is a true fact. The helmet can stimulate neural pathways causing altered states and/or hallucinations that have nothing to do with a religious practice or where God comes from.

You can stimulate the mind with drugs, such as LSD and other hallucinogenic drugs, that can do a similar thing. If you have a religious experience while taking the drug, that does not mean your brain created God. It should be noted that people with temporal lobe epilepsy report religious experiences. That doesn't mean that the temporal lobe forms God. The God spot in our brain is not the temporal lobe. The temporal lobe does have some association with religion and God, but it is not the source.

Rene Descartes was a seventeenth-century philosopher and scientist who wrote the book, *The Passions of the Soul*. He stated that the soul was located in the pineal gland. He described the pineal gland as, "a certain very small gland situated in the middle of the brain's substance and suspended above the passage through which the spirits in the brain's anterior cavities communicate with those in the posterior cavities."

Rick Strassman M.D., in his book called *The Spirit Molecule*, believes that the pineal gland is able to produce a hallucinogenic chemical called N-dimethyltryptamine (DMT), which he called the spirit molecule. This chemical causes a person to have mystical or psychedelic experiences. This may account for people having religious experiences. Again, there was no reliable follow up study by anyone independent, who saw the same results.

The pineal gland produces melatonin, which affects our sleep patterns in both seasonal and circadian rhythms. The pineal gland is the only midline structure in the brain. The name comes from the Latin word *pinea* which means its shape is like a pinecone. Some of the cells in the pineal gland (called *pinealocytes*) have the appearance of photoreceptor cells found in the retina of the eye. This is why it gets a lot of attention, as it has been called the third eye. Many people believe that this structure allows us to see into the spiritual world or is our connection to God. It still has an elevated status with people involved in psychospirituality and metaphysics.

The third eye is related to the Ajna chakra in eastern culture. The Hindus believe that the pineal gland is the third eye which they call the Eye of Dangma. It is called the all-seeing eye by the Buddists. There are references in Christianity of it being called the eye single. One of the largest pinecone sculptures in the world is in Vatican Square in the Court of the Pinecone. The pineal gland has been prominent in many cultures and philosophies throughout history. They believe that the pineal gland is the structure in the brain that leads them to their journey to spiritual enlightenment.

The pineal gland is only a gland that has cells similar to photoreceptor cells that produces melatonin during darkness and is inhibited by light. There is no solid reliable evidence that it does anything else. Some people take melatonin supplements for sleep.

Another interesting study printed in the *JAMA Psychiatry Journal* in February 2014 found that people who are religious have statistically significantly larger brains than non-religious people. It is not known why the brain is larger. It would indicate that brains of Christians are healthier. Having a relationship with God makes your brain larger and healthier. When your spirit connects with the Holy Spirit, your brain functions differently. As the Bible says, you are a new creature. In the study it was felt that larger brains had less instances of depression; or if the person did become depressed, it was milder and of shorter duration.

As I discussed in the chapter on the health benefits of a God-centered paradigm, Christians are healthier and live longer. It seems that atheists today are more militant than in the past. They are pushing their agenda into the lives of everyone. I bet that they are not happy about having smaller brains and not living as long.

In the book by Dean Hamer called *The God Gene*, he states that he has identified the gene that predisposes our level of spirituality. This gene is vesicular monoamine transporter 2 or VMAT2. It is a protein that covers or wraps chemical messengers in vesicles for transport through neurons in the brain.

When you are looking for reliable information from an author or researcher, you need to look at their background. Do they have a preset agenda? Is their research or opinions based narrowly only on a few bits of information and not viewed in the whole context of their study?

Are they open to learning about all the information available? Did they come to a different conclusion after their research?

There are excellent Christian books that provide great and reliable information. *Cold Case Christianity* by Jim Wallace, *The Case for Christ* by Lee Strobel, and *Seeking Allah, Finding Jesus* by Nabeel Qureshi are examples of where the facts led them to different conclusions than what they had in the beginning. Unfortunately, less than ten percent of scientists have a belief in God. That number seems to be changing recently, as prominent scientist, are producing work to show that science and religion can come to the same conclusion. *God of the Big Bang: How Modern Science Affirms the Creator* by Leslie Wickman, Ph.D. and *The Language of God: A Scientist Presents Evidence for Belief* by Francis Collins M.D. are examples. Douglas Axe has written a book called *Undeniable: How Biology Confirms our Intuition that Life is Designed*.

What do we know about our brains and how God affects our brains? As written in the chapter about how our brains work, we now have the capability of seeing what structures in the brain are active during a variety of activities. Functional MRIs can show activity in the brain, when a person is told to think or focus on a particular thought or activity. Single-photon emission computed tomography (SPECT) can also show where activity is located in the brain, when doing a specific activity. A radioisotope which emits gamma rays is injected into the blood stream through a vein. You ask the person to pray, meditate, or perform a particular activity. The radioisotope will collect more in an area with more activity. This can be captured with a gamma camera and provides a 3D image of the brain.

Dr. Andrew Newberg has done extensive study of the brain using these imaging systems. He has studied a variety of people: atheists, nuns, monks, Buddhists, Pentecostals speaking in tongues, and people who do extensive meditation daily.

What do these studies show about how God affects the brain? Is there a God spot in the brain? It turns out that there is not a God spot in the brain. The brain is much more complex than to have a single spot for God. As discussed earlier, the brain is extremely complex with billions of bits of data or information stimulating our senses. God has designed your brain so that you are able to connect with Him. God wants to be involved in your life. The Holy Spirit is connected to you throughout the complex network of neurons in your brain. Therefore, He has the ability to work in your brain to help guide you through life.

One point to make is, as I said earlier, it has been shown that Christians have larger brains. Dr. Andrew covers this in his book called *How God Changes Your Brain.* There are other researchers as well, such as Dr. Brick Johnstone. There must be something going on in the brain that is different in the brains of Christians. As discussed previously about Christians living longer and being healthier, maybe this better health contributes to the brain being larger and probably healthier. Or maybe the connection of your spirit to the Holy Spirit causes a change in the brain.

When people pray or concentrate on a religious experience, there are changes that occur in the brain. The prefrontal cortex becomes more active. This is the area that has to do with decision making, logic, attention, and intention. The anterior cingulate cortex is more active, as well. This area of the brain has to do with love, empathy, compassion, and helps to regulate our limbic system. There is reduced activity in the right posterior superior parietal lobe. One of the functions in this area of the brain is association. The parietal lobes help us orient ourselves to the world around us, especially in three-dimensional space. When people meditate, the parietal lobes become less active. People become less connected to themselves and more open to other things outside of themselves. Theoretically, this allows a person to sense or feel closer to God.

Dr. Johnstone studied twenty patients with traumatic brain injury to their right parietal lobes. People with this injury had an increased feeling of closeness to a higher power. Damage to this area decreases one's focus on self. This would indicate that religiosity or closeness to God is associated with a decreased focus on self, which makes sense. You have to turn your focus on God, Jesus, and/or the Holy Spirit in order to develop or experience God. This leads to self-transcendence or being connected to God.

Revelation 1:10 NLT

It was the Lord's Day and I was worshipping in the Spirit.

You can see John was *worshipping in the Spirit.* Spirit is capitalized, which means he was in direct association or communion with God. John was using the Sabbath as a day filled with worshipping God. He was taking this time seriously and purposefully. Real worship of God needs to be done in the appropriate manner. It appears that John was worshipping God through the Holy Spirit.

We have to assume that John's brain worked very similar to ours. Therefore, his frontal lobes and anterior cingulate cortex were actively involved with worshipping God. His right parietal lobe activity was diminished. He was focused on worshipping God and paying less attention to himself. This apparently is God's design for how our brain should work when we worship Him. John's mind was focused on God and not on his surroundings. He was connecting to the Holy Spirit through his spirit. This is an example of how we should worship God. You need to strive to use your brain in the manner that God has designed to worship Him. That doesn't mean that you should not take a couple of minutes at different times a day to reflect on God. But to gain a true closeness to God means spending quiet time with Him.

This is exactly what the teachings of Jesus are all about. You are to love God with all your heart, strength, mind, and soul. You are to love your neighbor as you love yourself. Christians are called to serve and put others first. You are happier and more fulfilled when giving rather than receiving. You may have heard a sermon about *a God-shaped hole in our hearts*. Our minds have a spirit that is longing or waiting to connect to God. It is only with that connection that man becomes complete and our brain increases in size—we become healthier and live longer.

With all this technology, we still don't know how the brain forms your consciousness, mind, thoughts, and beliefs; how your emotions are developed; or how your brain manages them. Let's take a look at what the Bible says about our minds and where we come from?

Ephesians 4:14-16 NLT

Then we will no longer be immature like children. We won't be tossed and blown about by every wind of new teaching. We will not be influenced when people try to trick us with lies so clever they sound like the truth. Instead, we will speak the truth in love, growing in every way more and more like Christ, who is the head of his body, the church. He makes the whole body fit together perfectly. As each part does its own special work, it helps the other parts grow, so that the whole body is healthy and growing and full of love.

It obviously will take time and effort to improve your ability to communicate to and with God. We will never understand everything about how your brain works. For every thought about God, there is a set of neurons that are firing in your brain. Every time a thought from the Holy Spirit pops up in your mind or you hear a voice advising you, there is a corresponding group of neurons firing. God communicates to you through the Holy Spirit inside your brain. The Holy Spirit is able to fire the appropriate neurons to communicate His thoughts to you. You worship by using specific brain cells that have been developed for this purpose. God is omnipotent. We will never fully know the extent of His power and majesty.

Romans 11:33-36 NLT

Oh, how great are God's riches and wisdom and knowledge! How impossible it is for us to understand his decisions and his ways! For who can know the Lord's thoughts? Who knows enough to give him advice? And who has given him so much that he needs to pay it back? For everything comes from him and exists by his power and is intended for his glory. All glory to him forever! Amen.

I know that we will never know all the answers to the mysteries of life. Science is continually advancing and many scientists are now seeing that our universe has been complexly and uniquely formed. This world didn't just happen by chance.

Romans 12:3 NLT

Because of the privilege and authority God has given me, I will give each of you a warning: Don't think you are better than you really are. Be honest in your evaluation of yourselves, measuring yourselves by the faith God has given us.

Philippians 3:15 NLT

Let us who are spiritually mature agree on these things. If you disagree on some point, I believe God will make it plain to you.

King Solomon wrote Ecclesiastes around the year 935 B.C. toward the end of his reign as King. At the time of King Solomon most people believed that the heart was the center of life, but King Solomon knew otherwise. His knowledge came from above. Look at what it says in Ecclesiastes.

Ecclesiastes 12:6-7 NLT

Yes, remember your Creator now while you are young, before the silver cord of life snaps and the golden bowl is broken. Don't wait until the water jar is smashed at the spring and the pulley is broken at the well. For then the dust will return to the earth, and the spirit will return to God who gave it.

This verse indicates that spirit and soul reside in the central nervous system. God breathed your spirit and soul into your central nervous system. As recorded in the Bible, we have the mind of Christ. God designed the central nervous system so that the Holy Spirit could reside in your brain or mind. That doesn't mean that the Holy Spirit isn't in every cell of your body. Your brain and mind are where you communicate with the Holy Spirit. Your spirit and soul are the source of life in your body.

The *silver cord of life* is the spinal cord, which is glistening and white while the person is alive. The *golden bowl* is the brain, which is bowl-like in shape and has a glistening yellowish-tan color. The term golden bowl and the silver cord of life also may be used here to refer to the preciousness of the contents of the brain. Solomon is saying that it is valuable like silver and gold. A bowl is a receptacle, which in this case is holding man's spirit and soul. The central nervous system being snapped from its attachment, indicates what happens when the soul and spirit leave the body—and the remaining body returns to dust. Another translation is that the spirit and soul are loosened from the body.

The body will die after this; the water and pulley are smashed or broken. Once the heart and its arteries stop pumping blood throughout the body, it begins to die. The spirit in the central nervous system is loosened and returned to God who gave it. God breathed into us our spirit and soul as, written in Genesis. Upon death the spirit returns to God.

Solomon's knowledge came from God. It is remarkable that he was able to describe the human body and life in the terms found in Ecclesiastes. At that time, man had no idea about the more complex functions of the body or where they were located. It wasn't until several hundred years later that Hippocrates stated that the brain was responsible for man's intelligence, thoughts, and soul. We now have the technology to study the brain during religious activities and have found out what parts of the brain are working while thinking, praying, meditating, or worshipping God.

I would like to close this chapter about where God is in the brain with a few observations. Our brains are extremely complicated, with millions of connections between different portions of the brain. It takes all of the different structures in the brain for us to live as we do.

- There is not a single specific spot in the brain for God. All the scientific evidence shows that multiple areas of the brain are involved in our relationship with God. God is not just in the temporal lobe or man does not have a single gene for God.
- There is no evidence that a gene or genes that man passes down from generation to generation to a structure in the brain creates God.
- Way before man had any knowledge of how the mind and body work, God told us through Solomon that our brain and central nervous system is where the Holy Spirit and man's spirit reside.
- That man has developed God out of fear of dying is not logical as many scientists have proposed. When was the last time that you had a mental crisis over the fear of dying?
- Christians have larger and healthier brains. In the past it was believed that the brain could not change after you grew up and matured. We now know that the brain is forming thousands of new neurons daily and your brain is constantly pruning unused neurons. Once the Holy Spirit enters your brain, you immediately start developing new neurons. Your mind goes through a transformation. I believe the Holy Spirit forms new neurons in your brain once He enters your mind.
- The Holy Spirit can keep forming new neurons as He needs them to communicate with you.

Isn't it great to know that God can make changes to your brain? This is the way the Holy Spirit communicates with you and helps guide you. For every thought about God, there is a corresponding set of neurons firing in your brain. The more time you spend thinking, praying, reading, and worshipping God, the more you form what I call *God neurons*. This is how you mature as a Christian. The more time you spend doing these things, results in less time you think about sinful things. Your stronger mind will have more control of your limbic system. Your brain will start to trim those bad neurons, as you are using them less. You start to have less stress, fear, worry, and anxiety. You are becoming a new creature, just like the butterfly coming from a caterpillar.

Read about God's invitation on living a God-centered paradigm found in Isaiah Chapter 55.

Isaiah Chapter 55 NLT

Is anyone thirsty? Come and drink—even if you have no money! Come, take your choice of wine or milk—it's all free! Why spend your money on food that does not give you strength? Why pay for food that does you no good? Listen to me, and you will eat what is good. You will enjoy the finest food. Come to me with your ears wide open. Listen, and you will find life. I will make an everlasting covenant with you. I will give you all the unfailing love I promised David. See how I used him to display my power among the peoples. I made him a leader among the nations. You will also command nations you do not know, and peoples unknown to you will come running to obey, because I, the Lord your God, the Holy One of Israel, have made you glorious." Seek the Lord while you can find him. Call on him now while he is near. Let the wicked change their ways and banish the very thought of doing wrong. Let them turn to the Lord that he may have mercy on them. Yes, turn to our God, for he will forgive generously. "My thoughts are nothing like your thoughts, "says the Lord. "And my ways are far beyond anything you could imagine."

God created us and our brains, not the other way around. God's Holy Spirit wants to be your partner in life. He wants to be your guide, instructor, and advocate. He wants to give you the fruits and gifts of the Spirit, and love you. He wants to be involved in everything you do.

He has designed your nervous system so that He can help you with your trials throughout life. All you have to do is decide to make God the priority in your life—and the possibilities become endless. If you have faith in Jesus Christ as Lord and Savior, the Holy Spirit will enter your mind and connect with your spirit.

Then, great things can happen!

Chapter 12
Work, Attitude, Success, and Winning

Luke 12:48 NLT
When someone has been given much, much will be required; and when someone has been entrusted with much, even more will be required.

Earlier in the book I discussed about how stress, anxiety, fear, and worry are the major cause of poor mental health and physical health. I stressed that you need to reduce or eliminate these from your life through developing a God-centered paradigm. And now I am going to tell you that you are called to work hard, have a positive cheerful attitude while working, and strive to win the race. How can you work hard and compete in a race without stress, anxiety, and worry? It all depends on your approach to life. The Bible is full of instructions about how you are to live your life, including your family and work.

There are surveys that show that nearly seventy-five percent of Americans have no sense of dignity or higher purpose in their jobs. Many people just punch the time clock and don't care about their job or how well they do it. I heard a story at an Order of St. Luke service about a lady who was there for prayer. The leader asked what she wanted to be prayed for and she stated she was having pain. She related that she was on disability for her chronic pain. The leader asked her if she wanted to be prayed for and healed of her pain. She said, "No! I don't want to be healed of my pain. If that occurred, I would lose my disability and would have to go back to work." The leader replied, "You would rather stay in pain and keep your disability, than go back to work pain free." She answered, "Yes." It's a shame that there are people who would rather live in misery and not participate in life, rather than be healthy living a full vibrant life.

Of course, there are people who love their work, people who hate their work, people who always complain about their work, people who try to avoid work, people who are lazy at their work, and people who only work because they have to work. The bottom line is that everyone needs to work. Your life on earth revolves around your work, where you live, when you sleep, when you eat, what you wear, the times you work, and the time you have vacation. Work is for a lifetime. God says in Genesis 3:19 that *by the sweat of your face shall you eat bread until you return to the ground.*

Let's take a look at what the Bible says about work, attitude, and winning.

God worked as He created the universe. He rested on the seventh day, not because He needed to rest, but to set an example for us to rest from our work and worship Him.

Genesis 2:1-3 NLT

So the creation of the heavens and the earth and everything in them was completed. On the seventh day God had finished his work of creation, so he rested from all his work. And God blessed the seventh day and declared it holy, because it was the day when he rested from all his work of creation.

God set an example of working, then resting on the Sabbath. He also placed man here to take care of His creation, which means you are to work for God to keep and maintain this world.

Genesis 1:26-30 NLT

Then God said, "Let's make human beings in our image, to be like us. They will reign over the fish in the sea, the birds in the sky, the livestock, all the wild animals on the earth, and the small animals that scurry along the ground."

So God created human beings in his own image. In the image of God he created them; male and female he created them. Then God blessed them and said, "Be fruitful and multiply. Fill the earth and govern it. Reign over the fish in the sea, the birds in the sky, and all the animals that curry along the ground." Then God said, "Look! I have given you every seed-bearing plant throughout the earth and all the fruit trees for your food. And I have given every green plant as food for all the wild animals, the birds in the sky, and the small animals that scurry along the ground—everything that has life." And that is what happened.

We are in charge and need to take care of His creation. God has called you to be His employee. There is nothing in the Bible that talks about retirement. You are to be His disciple for a lifetime. You are going to retire from your regular work, but living a Christian life is forever. In Ecclesiastes Chapter 2, it says that we are to enjoy food and drink and find satisfaction in work. Work is not a curse, but was ordained by God. By working hard with purpose, joyfully, honestly, diligently, enthusiastically, and with excellence, you are pleasing God.

Proverbs contains all kinds of verses about how to live our lives. Here are a few of them.

Proverbs 13:4 NLT

*Lazy people want much but get little,
but those who work hard will prosper.*

Proverbs 6:6-11 NLT

Take a lesson from the ants, you lazybones. Learn from their ways and become wise! Though they have no prince or governor or ruler to make them work, they labor hard all summer, gathering food for the winter. But you, lazybones, how long will you sleep? When will you wake up? A little extra sleep, a little more slumber, a little folding of the hands to rest—then poverty will pounce on you like a bandit; scarcity will attack you like an armed robber.

Proverbs 10:4-5 NLT

Lazy people are soon poor; hard workers get rich. A wise youth harvests in the summer, but one who sleeps during the harvest is a disgrace.

Proverbs 14:23-24 NLT

Work brings profit, but mere talk leads to poverty! Wealth is a crown for the wise; the effort of fools yields only foolishness.

1 Timothy 5:8 NLT

But those who won't care for their relatives, especially those in their household, have denied the true faith. Such people are worse than unbelievers.

Ecclesiastes 9:10 NLT

Whatever you do, do well.

Psalm 128:2 NLT

You will enjoy the fruit of your labor. How joyful and prosperous you will be!

Jeremiah 17:10 NLT

But I, the Lord, search all hearts and examine secret motives. I give all people their due rewards, according to what their actions deserve.

People who do not work hard and take their responsibility for themselves seriously will end up in poverty. Timothy states that people who don't care for their own relatives are worse than unbelievers. They are showing the world that Christians are no different or worse than unbelievers. You are like the moon reflecting light from God to others. As a Christian you are a representative of God and everything you do is a reflection of Him through you. If you love God and your family, you will make them a priority.

You are to prepare yourself for working in this world. In today's time that means getting an education and/or learning a vocation. If you fail to make the effort to do this, you are not following God's commands. Preparing your children for this world is your responsibility as a parent. The most important thing you can do is teach them about God and His instructions on life. Absolutely make sure that they get a great education. As a parent you cannot fail in your effort to make sure they are ready to go out on their own.

In your life and work you are to do everything to your best ability. There are people who suffer through hard times. They still need to persevere on and work to get themselves back on track. God does want us help them when they need help and God told us to take care of them.

Leviticus 23:22 NLT

When you harvest the crops of your land, do not harvest the grain along the edges of your fields, and do not pick up what the harvesters drop. Leave it for the poor and the foreigners living among you. I am the Lord your God.

One of the most rewarding things that I do is to provide care for people in need through the Bonita Springs Lions Eye Clinic. These people have no access to health care and are below poverty level. They don't even have Medicaid. The clinic provides free eye exams, glasses either at cost or free, and free surgery. Being able to help them has been extremely satisfying and rewarding. God calls us to help anyone in need. Take the time to work for a charity organization or an outreach program in your church. Christians should be taking care of their fair share of people in need, not just the government.

God also tells you to respect your bosses or companies that you work for. During the times that the Bible was written, slavery was common. God even goes as far as to tell us to be submissive to our masters. Obviously, we are all against any form of slavery; but no matter our work environment, believers in Christ should work hard and be a positive role model in the work place.

1 Peter 2:18-21 NLT

You who are slaves must submit to your masters with all respect. Do what they tell you—not only if they are kind and reasonable, but even if they are cruel. For God is pleased when, conscious of his will, you patiently endure unjust treatment. Of course, you get no credit for being patient if you are beaten for doing wrong. But if you suffer for doing good and endure it patiently, God is pleased with you. For God called you to do good, even if it means suffering, just as Christ suffered for you. He is your example, and you must follow his steps.

Wow, that is tough! Many times Christians have had to suffer and endure criticism, torture, and death because of their belief. In America, we are very fortunate to have freedom of religion. When you encounter problems at work, which everyone is going to encounter at some time, you need to approach it as an opportunity for Christian growth.

The people who suffer and endure these problems with the right attitude and approach will be blessed and honored by God. You are to follow in the steps of Christ.

As I am telling you about work ethic, there are other Bible verses that tell us how we should work.

Romans 12:11-12 NLT

Never be lazy, but work hard and serve the Lord enthusiastically. Rejoice in our confident hope. Be patient in trouble, and keep on praying.

2 Timothy 2:15 NLT

Work hard so you can present yourself to God and receive his approval. Be a good worker, one who does not need to be ashamed and who correctly explains the word of truth. Avoid worthless, foolish talk that only leads to more godless behavior.

God is telling you to be a hard worker. Christians should be the best employee at their work. He is also telling you that gossip and foolish talk is not good in the workplace. It only leads to bad things such as hurt feelings, poor work morale, and inferior work.

2 Thessalonians 3:6-13 NLT

And now, dear brothers and sisters, we give you this command in the name of our Lord Jesus Christ: Stay away from all believers who live idle lives and don't follow the tradition they received from us. For you know that you ought to imitate us. We were not idle when we were with you. We never accepted food from anyone without paying for it. We worked hard day and night so we would not be a burden to any of you. We certainly had the right to ask you to feed us, but we wanted to give you an example to follow. Even while we were with you, we gave you this command: "Those unwilling to work will not get to eat." Yet we hear that some of you are living idle lives, refusing to work and meddling in other people's business. We command such people and urge them in the name of the Lord Jesus Christ to settle down and work to earn their own living. As for the rest of you, dear brothers and sisters, never get tired of doing good.

God is telling you to stay away from people who are idle and do not work. They live on the backs of others. You know that there are many people who work the system to get their money from the government or other agencies. There is a culture in this country of people who choose not to work. Unfortunately, they pass this same culture down to the next generation. These people are not following the teaching and will of God.

In the beginning, God told Adam he was to work and take care of His garden. In my experience, people who work have a purpose in life and are happier. If people have set goals in their lives, they appear to enjoy life's journey. God designed and made you to work during your stay in this world. People are happiest when they are actively pursuing their goals. Just because you reach 65 does not mean that you back away from everything.

My church in Bonita Springs has a very large variance in attendance. The area population is extremely seasonal. In the winter, people from the north come to Florida for the winter. Many of them consider the time they spend in Florida as a vacation from life. They come to church on Sunday, but don't serve the church or community in any fashion. You should always continue forward with working for God and your community. After retirement, there should be much more time to spend on church related activities or other charities. You should always think about ways you can glorify God at work, play, and retirement.

What does the Bible say about how you should approach your work and what kind of attitude should you have?

Ephesians 6:7 NLT

Work with enthusiasm, as though you were working for the Lord rather than for people.

1 Corinthians 15:58 NLT

So, my dear brothers and sisters, be strong and immovable. Always work enthusiastically for the Lord, for you know that nothing you do for the Lord is ever useless.

You can see that God wants you to work enthusiastically at your work.

Philippians 2:14 NLT

Do everything without complaining and arguing, so that no one can criticize you. Live clean, innocent lives as children of God, shining like bright lights in a world full of crooked and perverse people.

Colossians 3:23-25 NIV

Whatever you do, work at it with all your heart, as working for the Lord, not for human masters, since you know that you will receive an inheritance from the Lord as a reward. It is the Lord Christ you are serving. Anyone who does wrong will be repaid for their wrongs, and there is no favoritism.

2 Corinthians 9:6-8 NLT

Remember this—a farmer who plants only a few seeds will get a small crop. But the one who plants generously will get a generous crop. You must decide in your heart how much to give. And don't give reluctantly or in response to pressure. "For God loves a person who gives cheerfully." And God will generously provide all you need. Then you will always have everything you need and plenty left over to share with others. As the Scriptures say, "They share freely and give generously to the poor. Their good deeds will be remembered forever."

Again, you are to be the best worker or employee. As a Christian, you are representing Christ to the world. You are to be a shining light reflecting God in you. Christians should work cheerfully, enthusiastically, diligently, honestly, with excellence, and knowing that everything you do is a reflection on God. While at work, perform your duties to the best of your abilities. After work, leave the work at work and go home to focus on God and family. You need to leave the stress, anxiety, and worry about anything concerning work at work.

Remember, you are to turn everything over to God—and that includes work. Trust in God that everything will work for your welfare. You need to help the less fortunate and provide for them with a portion of the blessings that God has provided for you. God wants a close relationship with you. Give him the time and focus on your part to make God the center of your paradigm. God is not telling you to be workaholic either.

Deuteronomy 8:18 NLT

Remember the Lord your God. He is the one who gives you power to be successful, in order to fulfill the covenant he confirmed to your ancestors with an oath.

Deuteronomy 30:9 NLT

The Lord your God will then make you successful in everything you do.

Matthew 6:19-34 NLT

*Don't store up treasures here on earth, where moths eat them and rust destroys them, and where thieves break in and steal.
Store your treasures in heaven, where moths and rust cannot destroy, and thieves do not break in and steal.
Wherever your treasure is, there the desires of your heart will also be.
Your eye is like a lamp that provides light for your body.*

*When your eye is healthy, your whole body is filled with light. But when your eye is unhealthy, your whole body is filled with darkness.
And if the light you think you have is actually darkness, how deep that darkness is! No one can serve two masters.
For you will hate one and love the other; you will be devoted to one and despise the other. You cannot serve God and be enslaved to money.*

That is why I tell you not to worry about everyday life—whether you have enough food and drink, or enough clothes to wear. Isn't life more than food, and your body more than clothing? Look at the birds. They don't plant or harvest or store food in barns, for your heavenly Father feeds them. And aren't you far more valuable to him than they are? Can all your worries add a single moment to your life? And why worry about your clothing? Look at the lilies of the field and how they grow. They don't work or make clothing, yet Solomon in all his glory was not dressed as beautifully as they are. And if God cares so wonderfully for wildflowers that are here today and thrown into the fire tomorrow, he will certainly care for you.

Why do you have so little faith? So don't worry about these things, saying, 'What will we eat? What will we drink? What will we wear?' These things dominate the thoughts of unbelievers, but your heavenly Father already knows your needs. Seek the Kingdom of God above all else, and live righteously, and he will give you everything you need. So don't worry about tomorrow, for tomorrow will bring its own worries. Today's trouble is enough for today.

You are not to let work dominate your life. If you are obsessed with work, your life will not be focused on God. Your family will suffer, as well. You have to trust that God will provide all that you need. Once you leave work, that part of your day is over. God wants to give everyone joy and peace.

As an ophthalmologist, I am particularly interested in verses 22 and 23. What you choose to see and focus on can completely control and/or influence your life. This is the basis of your paradigm. Your eye is like a lamp and provides light to your body. Who is the light of the world? Jesus is the light. If your paradigm is centered on Jesus, then His light will fill your body and soul. When your eye is healthy or focused on God, your whole body is filled with the light of the Holy Spirit. When your eye is unhealthy or your paradigm is not centered on God, your body is filled with darkness. As discussed in the chapter on health, non-Christians don't live as long. They have more mental and physical health issues. Once you are a child of God, you release all the anxiety, worry, stress, anger, and other negative feelings or thoughts. Jesus took all that on Himself on the cross.

What does our culture tell us about success? Remember the famous quote by Malcolm Forbes—*He who dies with the most toys wins.* Our culture today is obsessed with power, money, fame, fortune, prestige, and pleasure. Everyone wants everything right now. If you look at verses 19 to 21, you see that these things are just temporary. They are subject to decay and rust. None of these things can you take with you when you leave earth.

John Jacob Astor is quoted as saying, "I am the most miserable man on earth."

John D. Rockefeller stated, "I have made millions, but they brought me no happiness." What should you base your success on?

- Your success should be based on God's perspective.
- Have you followed the plan that God has for you?
- Have you been the best Christian possible?
- Is the world a better place because of the things you have done while on earth?
- Do you have a marriage based on Biblical principles?
- Did you raise your children in a Christian home?
- Does anyone who meets you know that you are a Christian? This is a saying that I like. (The deaf will hear and the blind will see that Christ is the center of your life).

There is a well-known parable in the Bible about how we should handle the gifts or money that God gives us in the parable of the three servants.

Matthew 25:14-30 NLT

Again, the Kingdom of Heaven can be illustrated by the story of a man going on a long trip. He called together his servants and entrusted his money to them while he was gone. He gave five bags of silver to one, two bags of silver to another, and one bag of silver to the last—dividing it in proportion to their abilities. He then left on his trip. The servant who received the five bags of silver began to invest the money and earned five more. The servant with two bags of silver also went to work and earned two more. But the servant who received the one bag of silver dug a hole in the ground and hid the master's money.

After a long time their master returned from his trip and called them to give an account of how they had used his money. The servant to whom he had entrusted the five bags of silver came forward with five more and said, 'Master, you gave me five bags of silver to invest, and I have earned five more.' The master was full of praise. 'Well done, my good and faithful servant. You have been faithful in handling this small amount, so now I will give you many more responsibilities. Let's celebrate together!

The servant who had received the two bags of silver came forward and said, 'Master, you gave me two bags of silver to invest, and I have earned two more.' The master said, 'Well done, my good and faithful servant. You have been faithful in handling this small amount, so now I will give you many more responsibilities. Let's celebrate together!'

Then the servant with one bag of silver came and said, 'Master, I knew you were a harsh man, harvesting crops you didn't plant and gathering crops you didn't cultivate. I was afraid I would lose your money, so I hid it in the earth. Look, here is your money back.' But the master replied, 'You wicked and lazy servant! If you knew I harvested crops I didn't plant and gather crops I didn't cultivate, why didn't you deposit my money in the bank? At least I could have gotten some interest on it.' The he ordered, 'Take the money from this servant, and give it to the one with the ten bags of silver.

To those who use well what they are given, even more will be given, and they will have abundance. But from those who do nothing, even what little they have will be taken away. Now throw this useless servant into outer darkness, where there will be weeping and gnashing of teeth.'

In some translations, the bag of silver is a talent. A talent is a Biblical measurement of weight which is usually applied to gold or silver. A talent was a considerable amount of money. In 1 Kings, a prison guard whose prisoner escaped would have been punished by death or he could pay a fine of one talent of silver. The master was letting these three men handle a significant amount of money. This parable shows us that we are responsible for what is given to us in this life. You are to manage it in a proper manner, so that it increases in value. You are asked to successfully manage your gifts and life.

Contrary to what is taught by many educators today, not all people are created with the same amount of talent (no pun intended). People will not all have the same amount of success or results. We are not rewarded equally. The people who work diligently and perform up to their capabilities will be more successful. God expects you to be a steward of the things He has given you in this life. In the end God is going to judge you on how you have lived your life. The third servant was judged for being lazy and not following his master's commands.

1 Kings 2:2-3 NLT

I am going where everyone on earth must someday go. Take courage and be a man. Observe the requirements of the Lord your God, and follow all his ways. Keep the decrees, command, regulations, and laws written in the law of Moses so that you will be successful in all you do and wherever you go.

David gave this advice to his son Solomon on how to be successful.

What does the Bible teach about winning? The Bible refers to a variety of athletic endeavors, competitions, and battles in relation to living our lives. Some of the verses talk about races or boxing. The Olympic Games were known in this period of time, as they first began in 776 B.C. on Mount Olympus. The beginning of the Olympics is said to have started by Herakles (not the more famous one who was the son of Zeus) and his four brothers. They raced at Mount Olympia to entertain the newborn Zeus.

The games continued every four years until the emperor Theodosius I stopped them in 394 A.D. as a campaign to impose Christianity as the state religion of Rome. There were probably a variety of games or sporting events scattered around that part of the world. Men have a tendency to show off their strength and skill!

Let's take a look at Bible verses about competition and winning with God's guidance and support.

2 Samuel 2:14 NIV

Then Abner said to Joab, "Let's have some young men get up and fight hand to hand in front of us."

Psalm 37:23-24 NLT

The Lord directs the steps of the godly. He delights in every detail of their lives. Though they stumble, they will never fall, for the Lord holds them by the hand.

Isaiah 40:31 NLT

But those who trust in the Lord will find new strength. They will soar high on wings like eagles. They will run and not grow weary. They will walk and not faint.

Ecclesiastes 9:10-11 NLT

Whatever you do, do well. I have observed something else under the sun. The fastest runner doesn't always win the race, and the strongest warrior doesn't always win the battle.

Philippians 3:13-14 NLT

But I focus on this one thing: Forgetting the past and looking forward to what lies ahead, I press on to reach the end of the race and receive the heavenly prize for which God, through Jesus Christ, is calling us.

Philippians 4:13 NLT

For I can do everything through Christ, who gives me strength.

Matthew 19:26 NLT

Jesus looked at them intently and said, "Humanly speaking, it is impossible. But with God everything is possible."

1 Timothy 4:7-8,12 NLT

Instead, train yourself to be godly. Physical training is good, but training for godliness is much better, promising benefits in this life and in the life to come. Don't let anyone think less of you because you are young. Be an example to all believers in what you say, in the way you live, in your love, your faith, and your purity.

2 Timothy 2:5 NLT

And athletes cannot win the prize unless they follow the rules.

2 Timothy 4:7-8 NLT

I have fought the good fight, I have finished the race, and I have remained faithful. And now the prize awaits me—the crown of righteousness, which the Lord, the righteous Judge, will give me on the day of his return. And the prize is not just for me but for all who eagerly look forward to his appearing.

Hebrews 12:1 NLT

Therefore, since we are surrounded by such a huge crowd of witnesses to the life of faith, let us strip off every weight that slows us down, especially the sin that so easily trips us up. And let us run with endurance the race God has set before us.

Hebrews 12: 11-13 NLT

No discipline is enjoyable while it is happening—it's painful! But afterward there will be a peaceful harvest of right living for those who are trained in this way. So take a new grip with your tired hands and strengthen your weak knees. Mark out a straight path for your feet so that those who are weak and lame will not fall but become strong.

The most competitive sports figure in the last several years was Tim Tebow. He played with a fierce competitive attitude. This attitude was transferred to his teammates. They played better when he was on the field. But when the game was over, he was a humble and mild-mannered Christian young man.

He gave all the glory of his success to Jesus Christ. He is a great example of how Christians should compete in this world. These are my favorite Bible verses about life, winning, and competition.

1 Corinthians 9:24-27 NLT

Don't you realize that in a race everyone runs, but only one person gets the prize? So run to win! All athletes are disciplined in their training. They do it to win a prize that will fade away, but we do it for an eternal prize. So I run with purpose in every step. I am not just shadowboxing. I discipline my body like an athlete, training it to do what it should.

These four Bible verses give us great instruction on how to live our lives. Whether it's a sporting event, race, or just everyday life, we are all participants. In sporting events, only one person will win the race and you should run the race to win. In life, everyone can win as the prize is the Kingdom of God. You should discipline yourself in your training. You should take every step forward with purpose. You are to approach life with a winning attitude. God calls you to be successful in the plan that He has for you and for every one of us. He wants you to reach the finish line, which occurs when you see Him in heaven.

What do the other Bible verses say about living your life? To win in life, it takes more than just physical abilities. It's about training, which at times may be painful and tedious. Winning also takes planning and preparation. Set goals for your life. You always do better if you have a goal to reach. You are to be cheerful and represent God to the world. There is a famous quote that says *You may be the only Bible that someone reads.* You are to live life, compete, and work enthusiastically, diligently, honestly, and be the best employee in the company. You are to play by the rules.

As it says in Philippians, you can do all things through Christ who strengthens you. You are to persevere and remain faithful. You have to believe you are going to win, to have any chance of winning. In a sport like basketball, if you don't believe one hundred percent that the shot you are taking is going in, your chances of making the shot are greatly diminished. The same goes for making a putt in golf. Now, you don't make them all, but you have to believe that you are going to make them all. In the end, you need to be able to say, "I have fought the good fight, I have finished the race, I have kept the faith."

I wrote this chapter because a friend of mine asked me what I thought about what someone said to him. They asked him how he was doing. He replied that he was doing well and everything was good. They told him that he should not say that he was doing great. Christians are supposed to be humble and not to boast. He wasn't sure how he should respond to this person.

That person was right about being humble and not boasting, but God has called us to be hard working successful people. You don't need to brag about how well you are doing, but you want others to see the peace, joy, happiness, success, and love in your life. If you aren't doing well, why would anyone who sees you want to become a Christian?

God gives instructions on living life in the Bible.

It is very clear that God is telling you, Bobby Di--------, Run to win!

Chapter 13
Emotions

Deuteronomy 7:7,9 NLT

The Lord did not set his heart on you and choose you because you were more numerous than the other nations, for you were the smallest of all nations! Understand, therefore, that the Lord your God is indeed God. He is the faithful God who keeps his covenant for a thousand generations and lavishes his unfailing love on those who love him and obey his commands.

Where do our emotions come from? We know that the limbic system located in our brain is where they originate in humans. I have stated earlier that our minds are modeled after God's mind according to the Bible. You see in the verse above that God has a heart. He has the emotion of love. So, your emotions are from God. You will find many references in the Bible about the emotions of God.

Are God's emotions the exact same as your emotions? Maybe, in some small way. God may use emotional terms in the Bible in a certain manner so that we can understand. If He does show emotions, they would be appropriate for the circumstance. Obviously, God is in total control of His emotions. Unfortunately, men and women have a tremendous amount of trouble controlling their emotions. We are all over the map, when it comes to our emotions. But, God is sovereign. He is the same yesterday, today, and tomorrow.

Faithfulness

Lamentations 3:22-23 NLT

The faithful love of the Lord never ends! His mercies never cease. Great is his faithfulness; his mercies begin afresh each morning.

Malachi 3:6 NLT

"I am the Lord, and I do not change."

Numbers 23:19 NLT

God is not man, so he does not lie. He is not human, so he does not change his mind.

The Bible verse at the beginning of the chapter in Lamentations also shows His faithfulness. God never changes and is always available. The Holy Spirit is present inside a Christian and is offering support 24/7.

Let's take a look some of the references to God's emotions in the Old Testament.

Compassion

Exodus 34:6-7 NLT

*The Lord passed in front of Moses, calling out,
Yahweh! The Lord! The God of compassion and mercy!
I am slow to anger and filled with unfailing love and faithfulness.
I lavish unfailing love to a thousand generations.
I forgive iniquity, rebellion, and sin.*

Nehemiah 9:19 NIV

Because of your great compassion you did not abandon them in the wilderness.

Even though the people of Israel turned from God time after time, he still showed them compassion. The NLT version of this verse uses the word *mercy* instead of compassion. I think these words have a very similar meaning. God is slow to anger which shows that He is in charge of His emotions. Many people have significant anger issues in this world. Your health, both physically and mentally, would be much better if you control your anger. The constant release of the fight and fright chemicals into your body is very harmful. Let God show you how to control your anger, if you have problems dealing with it.

Jealousy

The word in the Old Testament for *jealous* means to become intensely red. This refers to the changing in color of the face. It can also mean the rising of heat emotionally. It means intense zeal or fervor over something dear to a person. In the New Testament the word for *jealousy* is translated many times as zeal. God is a jealous God. We are to worship Him and no other God. The second of the Ten Commandments is: *You must not have any other god but me.* God is also telling you to love with passion, conviction, and zeal.

Exodus 34:14 NLT

You must worship no other gods, for the Lord, whose very name is Jealous, is a God who is jealous about his relationship with you.

Laughing

Psalm 2:4 NLT

But the one who rules in heaven laughs.

Joy

Nehemiah 8:10 NLT

And Nehemiah continued, "Go and celebrate with a feast of rich foods and sweet drinks, and share gifts of food with people who have nothing prepared. This is a sacred day before our Lord. Don't be dejected and sad, for the joy of the Lord is your strength!"

Love

I devoted a chapter on God's love, as this is the cornerstone of life. In the New Testament, life was condensed down to two commandments.

We are to love God with all our heart, soul, strength, and mind. We are to love our neighbor as yourself. As I have said before, if we all did this, most of the world's problems would vanish.

God also has some emotions that you might consider negative, such as, anger, vengeance, hate, and wrath.

These emotions are related to God's response to man's sins and man's continual turning away from Him. These emotions are also toward non-believing people, especially those who have done things against his chosen people. God cannot and does not tolerate sin or worship of other gods.

Wrath, Vengeance, Revenge

This was God's message for Philistia, who acted against Judah out of bitter revenge and long-standing contempt.

Ezekiel 25:17 NLT

I will execute terrible vengeance against them for what they have done. And when I have inflicted my revenge, they will know that I am Lord.

Other translations include the word *wrath*. God does react to man's transgressions with emotion.

Hate, Detest, Abhor, Despise

Leviticus 20:23 NLT

Do not live according to the customs of the people I am driving out before you. It is because they do these shameful things that I detest them.

Leviticus 26:30 NLT

I will destroy your pagan shrines and knock down your places of worship. I will leave your lifeless corpses piled on top of your lifeless idols, and I will despise you.

Psalm 5:5-6 NLT

Therefore, the proud may not stand in your presence, for you hate all who do evil. You will destroy those who tell lies. The Lord detests murders and deceivers.

Next, let's see what the Bible says about Jesus' emotions. Did Jesus have to deal with the same emotions that you deal with? He had a limbic system, just as you do. Therefore, He had to deal with His emotions everyday, just like you and I.

Philippians 2:6-8 NLT

Though he was God, he did not think of equality with God as something to cling to. Instead, he gave up his divine privileges; he took the humble position of a slave and was born as human being. When he appeared in human form, he humbled himself in obedience to God and died a criminal's death on a cross.

Jesus, being both God and man, did have and experience emotions. Different from us, His emotions were perfect for each instance in His life. He had to deal with His limbic system. His limbic system (just like yours) did produce emotions, but with God they were perfect for each situation. Jesus was able to be in complete control. Obviously, His Spirit was able to control His limbic system and was able to be in total control of His physical nature. Hebrews confirms that He had the same temptations and had to control His limbic system.

Pain and Suffering

Hebrews 4:14-15 NLT

So then, since we have a great High Priest who has entered heaven, Jesus the Son of God, let us hold firmly to what we believe. This High Priest of ours understands our weaknesses, for he faced all of the same testings we do, yet he did not sin.

This next verse relates back to the basis of this book and the chapter on Paradigms in the Bible. Jesus was not recognized by His own people, which was foretold in Isaiah. He felt the pain and suffering during His ministry. Jesus most assuredly felt the physical pain and the pain of taking all of mankind's sins onto Himself on the cross. That pain is beyond our comprehension.

Isaiah 53:4 NLT

*Surely he took up our pain and bore our suffering,
yet we considered him punished by God,
stricken by him, and afflicted.*

Compassion

Luke 7:12-15 NLT

A funeral procession was coming out as he approached the village gate. The young man who had died was a widow's only son, and a large crowd from the village was with her. When the Lord saw her, his heart overflowed with compassion. "Don't cry!" he said. Then he walked over to the coffin and touched it, and the bearers stopped. "Young man," he said, "I tell you, get up." Then the dead boy sat up and began to talk! And Jesus gave him back to his mother.

Matthew 9:36 NLT

When Jesus saw the crowds, he had compassion on them because they were confused and helpless, like sheep without a shepherd.

Matthew 11:28-30 NLT

Then Jesus said, "Come to me, all of you who are weary and carry heavy burdens, and I will give you rest. Take my yoke upon you. Let me teach you, because I am humble and gentle at heart, and you will find rest for your souls. For my yoke is easy to bear, and the burden I give you is light."

Just as in the Old Testament where God is found to have a heart or soul, Jesus has a heart and soul. He has a human heart or soul and a God heart or soul. Jesus loves and has compassion when He sees people who are grieving or needing help.

Love

Mark 10:21 NLT

Looking at the man, Jesus felt genuine love for him. "There is still one thing you haven't done," he told him. "Go and sell all your possessions and give the money to the poor, and you will have treasure in heaven. Then come, follow me."

The story of Lazarus shows how much Jesus loved His followers. Jesus was troubled and emotional as He observed His friends and followers. It moved Him so much that He wept or cried.

John 11: 33-36 NLT

When Jesus saw her weeping and saw the other people wailing with her, a deep anger welled up within him, and he was deeply troubled. "Where have you put him?" he asked them. They told him, "Lord, come and see." Then Jesus wept. The people who were standing nearby said, "See how much he loved him!"

Joy

Jesus felt joy just like we can feel joy. In fact, He wants to give us a special joy that can only come from God.

John 15:11 NLT

I have told you these things so that you will be filled with my joy. Yes, your joy will overflow!

Wept or Crying

The shortest verse in the Bible is in John.

John 11:35 NIV

Jesus wept.

The next Bible verse is about Jesus weeping, but it also is related to paradigms in the Bible. Jesus understands that His people still do not understand what is going to happen. They are cheering Him as He approaches the city; but he knows that in a few short days, they are going to crucify Him. The word for wept here is *klaio,* which not only means to weep or cry but to show outward grief or mourning.

Luke 19:41 NLT

As he approached Jerusalem and saw the city, he wept over it and said, If you, even you, had only known on this day what would bring you peace—but now it is hidden from your eyes.

Sorrow, Despair

Matthew 27:46 NLT

About three in the afternoon Jesus cried out in a loud voice. "Eli, Eli, lema sabachthani?" (which means "My God, my God, why have you forsaken me?").

As an interesting side note. Jesus also appears to be referring to Psalm 22. His statement is the first verse of Psalm 22 that talks about His crucifixion.

Anger, Sadness

He looked at them angrily and was deeply saddened by their hard hearts.

Matthew 21:12-13 NLT

Jesus enters the Temple and began to drive out all the people buying and selling animals for sacrifice. He knocked over the tables of the money changers and the chairs of those selling doves. He said to them, "The Scriptures declare, 'My Temple will be called a house of prayer,' but you have turned it into a den of thieves!"

Jesus did have what we might think of as a negative emotion of anger, but it was appropriate for the setting. His house had been turned into a den of thieves, sinners. He became upset that His people would do such a thing in this Holy place.

Anguish

Luke 22:44 NLT

He prayed more fervently, and he was in such agony of spirit that his sweat fell to the ground like great drops of blood.

Sweating blood or hematidrosis is a very rare clinical phenomenon in which a person sweats blood. The blood usually comes from the forehead, umbilicus or belly button, nails, nosebleeds, blood stained tears, and other skin surfaces. There are two major causes. It may occur with certain systemic diseases, excessive exertion, bleeding disorders, psychogenic, and unknown factors. The other cause is severe mental anxiety or stress. As the anxiety increases, the blood vessels or capillaries that surround the sweat glands rupture. The blood enters the sweat glands and is pushed along with sweat to the surface. There have been reports of soldiers who sweated blood before a battle. Jesus experienced such extreme anguish, anxiety, and stress in the Garden of Gethsemane that He sweated blood. It is very evident that Jesus experienced emotion.

There are many other verses that show the different emotions that Jesus displayed. The difference is that Jesus was in control of His emotions. His Spirit and soul were able to keep His limbic system in perfect control. The goal of everyone should be to be as much like Jesus as possible.

The closer you can come to being like Jesus, the more control you will have over your negative emotions. The Holy Spirit inside of you will help your soul control your limbic system. You are to model yourself after Jesus.

1 John 2:6 NIV

Whoever claims to live in him must live as Jesus did.

Philippians 2:1-5 NIV

Therefore, if you have any encouragement from being united with Christ, if any comfort from his love, if any common sharing in the Spirit, if any tenderness and compassion, then make my joy complete by being like-minded, having the same love, being one in spirit and one mind. Do nothing out of selfish ambition or vain conceit. Rather, in humility value others above yourselves, not looking to your own interests but each of you to the interests of the others. In your relationships with one another, have the same mindset as Christ Jesus.

1 Peter 2:21-23 NLT

He is your example, and you must follow his steps. He never sinned, nor ever deceived anyone. He did not retaliate when he was insulted, nor threaten revenge when he suffered. He left his case in the hands of God.

As you see from the Scriptures, it is okay to have emotions, as you get them from God. Your emotions are God's gift to you. Emotions add a richness to your life. The problem for many people is that their emotions become so intense that it alters who they are. Their out of control emotions dominant their lives. It causes many negative things. You cannot flee from your emotions, as they are a part of you. But, you need to learn how to keep your emotions at a healthy level.

There are good, happy, or joyful emotions and negative emotions. Negative emotions are normal, but you need to harness them. Do not let them get out of control and their duration needs to be limited, in order for the brain to function at its optimum level. As discussed in prior chapters, negative emotions cause physical and mental diseases.

Emotions make life enjoyable. The key is to express your emotions, as Jesus expressed His emotions. Handle your emotions by developing a close relationship with the Holy Spirit. The Holy Spirit has emotions as well, but the Holy Spirit is in control of His emotions. One of the Holy Spirit's main functions is to guide you through the daily emotions of life. The Holy Spirit is ready to fill your emotional life with joy, peace, happiness, and love. The Holy Spirit gives the fruits and gifts revealed in the Bible, which were covered in earlier chapters. Read Colossians Chapter 3 which talks about living out life. Here is a short synopsis.

- Set your sights on the realities of heaven.
- Think about things of heaven.
- Put to death or stop thinking about the earthly sins lurking inside you.
- Stop sexual immorality, impurity, lust, and evil desires.
- Don't be greedy and worship the things of the world.
- Get rid of anger, rage, malicious behavior, slander, lying, and dirty language.
- Clothe yourself with tenderhearted mercy, kindness, humility, gentleness, and patience.
- Let peace rule your heart and clothe yourself with love.
- Teach and counsel each other.
- Let the message of Christ fill your life.
- Whatever you do or say, you are doing as a representative of the Lord Jesus.

The Holy Spirit, full of love and emotion, is in your brain. The Spirit is intertwined with your spirit and soul. The Holy Spirit is sending you signals, instructions, advice, trying to stop the bad emotions or influences in your mind, and activating neurons in your brain stimulating positive emotions to live by.

Be emotional for God!

Chapter 14
Meditation

Psalm 46:10 NLT
Be still, and know that I am God!

Psalm 62:1 NLV
My soul is quiet and waits for God alone.
He is the One Who saves me.

I realize that meditation is a touchy subject for many Christians. But, you need to be careful when you decide that something is bad without researching what the Bible says about it. We are told to meditate more than twenty times in the Bible. I know that most people associate meditation with Eastern traditions or mysticism, such as Buddhism and Hinduism. These practices are associated with transcending the mind or brain to an alignment or enlightenment in the world or cosmos. Transcendental meditation was created by Maharishi Mahesh Yogi of the Hindu religion, which is based on Hindu philosophy. What these traditions do in their meditation, should not influence what a Christian should be doing in their Christian life and walk with God.

Christian meditation is based on developing a closer relationship with God and obtaining a deeper or better understanding of the Bible. I will also show you that you can improve your brain function with the proper meditation. So not only will you develop a closer relationship with God, but you can improve your brain function, as well. If there are central nervous system diseases such as Alzheimer's in your family history, this very important to you.

What is Christian meditation? Christian meditation is a form of prayer. It is a mental exercise of focusing attention, relaxing the mind, and calming the body. It is a time to reflect, study, pray, and read God's Word. Christian meditation is focused on God and is designed to stimulate thought and understanding. Christian meditation is distinctly different from Eastern forms of meditation. In Christian meditation, you are to fill and focus your mind on God or God's Word, compared to emptying or disengaging your mind in the Eastern forms of meditation.

In the Old Testament, there are two Hebrew words that are used for meditation. The first word is *haga* which means to sigh, murmur, or meditate. The second word *siha* means to muse or rehearse in one's mind. The Greek word for meditate is *melete*. This word emphasizes meditation movements in the depth of the heart. The Latin word is *meditatio*. Many times when the word meditation appears in the Bible, it is followed by a verse on obedience.

Definition of meditate in *The Free Dictionary* is:
- To train, calm, or empty the mind, often by achieving an altered state, as by focusing on a single object, especially as a form of religious practice in Buddhism or Hinduism.
- To engage in devotional contemplation, especially prayer.
- To think about something deeply.
- To reflect deeply on spiritual matters, especially as a religious act.
- To plan, consider, or think of doing.
- To engage in thought or contemplation.

Meditation

Synonyms: Mull, muse, ponder, think over, reflect, cogitate, cerebrate, theologize, introspect, consider, deliberate, ruminate, study, chew on, explore, grapple, reason, reckon, turn over, wonder, and wrestle with.

A lot of the controversy with Christian meditation is that through history there have been many forms of meditation. Meditation falls into the category of contemplative practice. There are three forms of Christian contemplative practice.

- Contemplative prayer involves the silent repetition of sacred words or sentences with focus and devotion.

- Contemplative reading involves thinking deeply about teaching or events in the Bible.

- Sitting with God is a silent meditation; this is usually preceded by contemplative prayer or reading. You focus your mind, soul, and heart on God.

There numerous types of meditation around the world and throughout history.

The famous evangelist Charles Spurgeon stated, "The Spirit has taught us in meditation to ponder its message, to put aside, if we will, the responsibility of preparing the message we've got to give. Just trust God for that."

Hesychasm (Eastern Orthodox) or Jesus Prayer began in the desert of the Middle East and means stillness or silence. There are the spiritual exercises of Saint Ignatius of Loyola. He was the founder of the Jesuits who wrote Spiritual Exercises. These meditation methods are still used by the Roman Catholic Church's religious order of Jesuits. Some of these methods involve imagery, such as imagining being present at one of the events discussed in the Bible. Imagine yourself talking with Jesus and asking Him questions.

Another famous leader in the church was St. Teresa of Avila. She was a proponent of contemplative prayer or meditation. She taught the nuns that meditation was a process of being in communion with God. She wrote several books about prayer and meditation.

Saint Thomas Aquinas believed that meditation is a necessary component for devotion. The rosary is a form of meditation.

Another form of Christian meditation that has been used since the fourth century is *Lectio Divina*. Lectio Divina means divine word or reading. This has four stages of progression.

- The reading stage begins with finding a Bible verse and reading it deliberately.
- The second stage is called discursive meditation where you think and cogitate on the passage.
- The third stage is effective prayer, as you pray to God about the text and ask Him to reveal to you the meaning of the passage.
- The fourth stage is contemplation where you simply remain quiet and still in God's presence.

There many forms of Christian meditation. Even a short simple prayer is a form of meditation. The regular practice of Christian meditation helps to change your paradigm towards one that is centered on God. Christian meditation is Christ or God-centered. King David delighted in meditating on God day and night.

I am going to focus on simple meditation practices that are going to be based on God and the Bible. I will also give you scientific evidence that shows you can change the manner in which your brains functions and that it will improve your cognitive abilities. So this meditation practice that I am going to recommend to you will bring you closer to God and improve your brain as well. This is a win, win!!

Thomas Merton who was an American Catholic writer and Trappist monk believed that Christian meditation's goal is: *The true end of Christian meditation is practically the same end of liturgical prayer and the reception of the sacraments: a deeper union by grace and charity with the Incarnate Word, who is the only Mediator between God and man, Jesus Christ.* One of the main goals of Christian meditation is to worship and bring joy to the heart of God. Meditation shows God that we love Him through obedience, honor, and adoration.

E. P. Clowney, who was an ordained pastor in the Orthodox Presbyterian Church, described Christian meditation as having three dimensions.

- The first dimension is that Christian meditation is grounded on the Bible. Because the God of the Bible is a personal God who speaks in words of revelation, Christian meditation responds to this revelation and focuses on that aspect. This is in contrast to mystic meditations which use mantras.
- The second dimension of Christian meditation is that it responds to the love of God. This love of God is the cornerstone of Christian communion and is increased by Christian meditation.
- The third dimension is the revelation of the Bible and the love of God leading to the worship of God; making Christian meditation an exercise in praise.

Jim Downing, who wrote the book *Meditation*, states that God considers meditation *a vital exercise of the minds of His children.*

Saint Padre Pio, who was a strong believer in rosary meditations, stated, "The person who meditates and turns his mind to God, who is the mirror of his soul, seeks to know his faults, tries to correct them, moderates his impulses, and puts his conscious in order."

Dr Bruce Demarest, who is a faculty member of the Denver Seminary, wrote, *A quieted heart is our best preparation for all this work of God… Meditation refocuses us from ourselves and from the world so that we reflect on God's word, His nature, His abilities, and His works… So* we prayerfully ponder, muse, and 'chew' the words of scripture... *The goal is simply to permit the Holy Spirit to activate the life-giving Word of God.*

Rick Warren of Saddleback Church and author of *The Purpose Driven Life* states in the book that *Meditation is focused thinking. It takes serious effort. You select a verse and reflect on it over and over in your mind... if you know how to worry, you already know how to meditate.* He also states that *No other habit can do more to transform your life and make you more like Jesus than daily reflection on Scripture... If you look up all the times God speaks about meditation in the Bible, you will be amazed at the benefits He has promised to those who take the time to reflect on His Word throughout the day.*

Are Christians supposed to mediate? Let's see what the Bible says about meditation.

Genesis 24:63 ESV

And Isaac went out to meditate in the field toward evening.

Joshua 1:8 NLT

Study this Book of Instruction continually. Meditate on it day and night so you will be sure to obey everything written in it. Only then will you prosper and succeed in all you do.

Psalm 1:2 NLT

But they delight in the law of the Lord, meditating on it day and night.

Psalm 19:14 NLT

May the words of my mouth and the meditation of my heart be pleasing to you, O Lord, my rock and my redeemer.

Psalm 49:3 ESV

My mouth shall speak wisdom, the meditation of my heart shall be understanding.

Psalm 104:34 ESV

May my meditation be pleasing to him, for I rejoice in the Lord.

Psalm 119:15 NIV

I will meditate on your precepts and consider your ways.

Psalm 119:27 NLT

Help me understand the meaning of your commands, and I will meditate on your wonderful deeds.

Psalm 119:48 NIV

I reach out for your commands, which I love, that I may meditate on your decrees.

Psalm 119:97 ESV

Oh how I love your law! It is my meditation all the day.

Psalm 119:148 NIV

My eyes stay open through the watches of the night, that I may meditate on your promises.

Philippians 4:8 NLV

Christian brothers, keep your minds thinking about whatever is true, whatever is respected, whatever is right, whatever can be loves, and whatever is well thought of. If there is anything and worth giving thanks for, think about these things.

1 Timothy 4:15 KJV

Meditate upon these things; give yourself wholly to them; that thy profiting may appear to all.

Philippians 4:8-9 NLT

And now, dear brothers and sisters, one final thing. Fix your thoughts on what is true, and honorable, and right, and lovely, and admirable. Think about things that are excellent and worthy of praise. Keep putting into practice all you have learned and received from me—everything you heard from me and saw me doing. Then the God of peace will be with you.

These Bible verses tell us that we should meditate on God's words, commands, precepts, and promises. We are to do it, because it pleases God's heart. It will help you prosper, succeed, and make you a better witness to others. Meditation calls out upward toward God. We are to connect with God through His Holy Spirit and our spirit. Then your heart and soul will be filled with love, joy, happiness, and peace. You will gain wisdom and understanding. You will be able to comprehend what the plans are that God has for your life.

There is no question that we are to meditate on God and His Word. The key is that we need to do it in a Christian manner. What other traditions or religions choose to do, should having nothing to do with following the teachings of God's Word.

As I said earlier, meditation can physically change the way your brain functions. Not only does meditation benefit your spiritual life, but it helps your brain work in a more efficient and balanced way. Let's take a look the different ways meditation improves your mental and physical health.

Brain and Mental Improvements with Meditation
- Decreases the incidence of depression and dysfunctional thinking.
- Reduces stress, anger, and anxiety.
- Helps control or regulate anxiety and mood.
- Helps control panic disorders.
- Improves the health and thickness of the brain.
- Improves prefrontal cortex processing and decision making.
- Improves the ability to stay focused and work under stress.
- Improves the severity of pain.
- Improves learning, memory, and rapid memory recall.
- Improves your visuospatial processing in the parietal lobe.

- Increases compassion.
- Decreases worry.
- Improves relationships.

Health

- Reduces blood pressure.
- Reduces the risk of heart attacks and strokes.
- Improves your immune system.
- Decreases inflammatory diseases such as rheumatoid arthritis, fibromyalgia, inflammatory bowel disease, and others.
- Reduces the risk of Alzheimer's disease and other degenerative brain diseases.

As you can see, meditation improves a significant number of disorders and diseases. Just from a medical standpoint, everyone should meditate every day. Meditation reduces anxiety, worry, stress, anger, and depression. Meditation reduces blood pressure, heart rate, controls the release of stress hormones, reduces heart attacks, and strokes. Meditation helps with the things discussed in the health chapter about living a healthier and longer life. Meditation has been shown to improve cognitive brain function and helps prevent diseases of the brain like Alzheimer's disease.

It is possible to exercise and train your mind through a variety of techniques. For those who are opposed to any type of Eastern-like meditation, you don't have to follow their methods. Meditation and the other techniques that I am going to describe are based on research and science. I am going to use the scientific research and combine it with a Christian based system. One of the main purposes of this book is to help you change your paradigm or life and make it more centered on God. It is to show you how to have a closer relationship with the Triune God.

Dr. Andrew Newberg has written several books on God and the brain. The book, *How God Changes Your Brain,* is a great book filled with significant amount of scientific information. He gives eight ways or steps for you to perform so you can improve your brain activity, based on functional MRIs, PET scans, SPECT scans, and other research. If you are interested in learning more about how God works in your brain, read his books.

8. Smile—just smiling repetitively interrupts mood disorders and strengthens the brain's neural processes.

7. Stay intellectually active.

6. Consciously relax.

5. Yawn—According to Dr. Newberg, yawning is one of the best kept secrets in neuroscience. Several recent brain scan studies have shown that yawning evokes a unique neural activity in the areas of the brain, that are directly involved with generating social awareness and creating feelings of empathy.

4. Meditate—When it comes to enhancing spiritual experiences, it takes first place. Even ten to fifteen minutes of meditation appears to have significantly positive effects on cognition, relaxation, and psychological health.

3. Aerobic exercise—Forty-five minutes of a cardiovascular workout every other day is enough to keep your brain healthy.

2. Dialogue with others.

1. Faith—provides hope, optimism, and the belief that a positive future awaits us.

As I discussed previously, Christians live longer and have less depression.

Dr. Newberg has done numerous studies. His study on a particular meditation technique had significant changes in the brain.

This meditation technique increases activity in the prefrontal cortex and anterior cingulate, which improves memory and cognition. At the end of twelve minutes of meditation, there is decreased activity in the parietal lobes, which is the part of the brain you use to orient yourself or have a sense of self awareness. This change in activity in the parietal lobe prepares your mind, so that it can better sense what you are meditating on.

Meditation has been shown to counter the effects of depression. Parkinson's and Alzheimer's patients have reduced metabolic activity in the anterior cingulate. Personal religious practices and higher levels of spirituality are associated with slower progression of Alzheimer's disease. Brief prayer has not shown to have a direct effect on cognition. When prayer is incorporated into longer forms of intense meditation or practiced within the context of weekly religious activity, many health benefits have been found.

In one study of meditation, the brain-scan showed a strengthening in a specific circuit in the brain. This circuit involved the prefrontal and orbital-frontal lobe, the anterior cingulate, basal ganglia, and thalamus. This circuit governs a wide variety of activities involved with consciousness, clarity of mind, reality formation, error detection, empathy, compassion, emotional balance and the suppression of anger and fear. The study also showed increased activity in the basal ganglia which help control voluntary movements, posture, and motor sequencing. It also is involved in memory formation, behavioral control, and cognitive flexibility.

Abnormal functioning in these areas are associated with normal aging, Parkinson's, Alzheimer's, Tourette's, and Huntington's disease. There is also decreased activity in the parietal lobe which regulates our sense of self. This meditation technique was only twelve minutes long and included movements as well. It appears that movement-based meditation strengthens the parts of the brain susceptible to many age-related diseases. One of the patients in this study improved their cognitive abilities by almost fifty percent in less than four months!

Here are my recommendations for preparing to develop a meditation routine. Since over fifty percent of brain is used for receiving and processing sensory input, it is logical that you involve your senses during your meditation. You need to create an environment that promotes the quality of your time meditating and spending time with God. You should find a quiet place and a comfortable chair. You may wish to light a candle. Remember that Jesus is the light of the world. You should consider playing Christian instrumental music softly in the background. Christian instrumental music provides a quiet place for hearing God's voice and connecting with Him. It provides support for your prayer and worship. A good source for this can be found on line at www.secretplaceministries.org .

You may wish to use a daily devotional as the source for your Scripture reading. There are many of those available. You need to choose a time in the day that you can set aside approximately thirty minutes. I believe that early in the morning is a great time. It is also a great way to start your day and center your life for the day on God. If you have children that you need to get ready for school early in the morning, then after they go to bed at night is ok as well.

Meditation Steps:

Prepare the room as you choose to do: light your candle, start the background music, get your Bible and daily devotional materials by your chair.

- Sit in a comfortable chair.
- Calm yourself, yawn four or five times, take three or four slow deep breathes through your nose. (Breathing through your nose raises the nitric oxide in your body, which increases blood flow to the brain by dilating the blood vessels.)

Meditation

- Begin by touching your thumb to each finger in succession on one hand then the other. Either say out loud, whisper, or silently think the words—God, Jesus, Holy Spirit—as you touch each finger beginning on one hand and then the other. You can use other words relating to God, if you wish. Do this for ten minutes. (You should set a timer, so that you do not have to think about when your ten minutes are up. Your smart phone will do fine.)
- Stop, be still, and listen to your mind and soul for a minute.
- Try to listen for your spirit in communication with the Holy Spirit.
- Pick up your Bible or daily devotional. Read the text that you have chosen.
- Stop, be still, and contemplate what the passage is saying to you. Read it a second time, if you need to read or hear the words again.
- Think about asking yourself the questions I discussed about evaluating an event: what, when, where, why, who, and etc. If the Bible verse is about a particular event, place yourself there and see if you perceive or understand it in a different manner. See how many different viewpoints you can think about relating to the Bible verse, in what context, and other nuances.
- Practice perceiving or seeing through God-centered eyes. Strengthen your spiritual vision.
- Pray.
- Be still and know that I am God.
- Keep a journal of your thoughts and experiences.

The health and spiritual benefits can be amazing. If you don't feel comfortable calling it meditation, think of this as your devotional time, just simple prayer, or quiet time with God. Rhonda Jones has written instructional guide called *A Date with God*. That's a great way of thinking about it. She believes that it is like a daily shower for the soul.

Start your day believing that Jesus is at your side all day. He is there in the form of the Holy Spirit). He is your wing man or your partner for life. If someone cuts you off in traffic and Jesus was driving, what would He do? If you encounter a rude person, what would Jesus do? You are in entering the checkout line and someone cuts in front of you, what would Jesus say or do? Try living your life each day thinking that way. You should be able to complete your meditation in thirty minutes or less.

This meditation practice will enhance your relationship to God. It will strengthen the connection of your spirit and the Holy Spirit. This will help your soul keep its focus on God and maintain control over your limbic system. Your brain will function in a more efficient and balanced manner. You may delay the onset of many degenerative neurological diseases.

1 Chronicles 28:9 NLT

And Solomon, my son, learn to know the God of your ancestors intimately. Worship and serve him with your whole heart and a willing mind. For the Lord sees every heart and knows every plan and thought. If you seek him, you will find him.

I hope that you see that meditation is an important part of being a Christian and connecting to God. It will change your paradigm.

It has benefits for you spiritually, mentally, and physically.

God wants to spend quality time with you!

Chapter 15
A God-Centered Paradigm (Life)
Place Your Life Before God

Romans 12:1-2 MSG

So here's what I want you to do, God helping you: Take your everyday, ordinary life—your sleeping, eating, going-to-work, and walking-around life—and place it before God as an offering. Embracing what God does for you is the best thing you can do for him. Don't become so well-adjusted to your culture that you fit into it without even thinking. Instead, fix your attention on God. You'll be changed from the inside out. Readily recognize what he wants from you, and quickly respond to it. Unlike the culture around you, always dragging you down to its level of immaturity, God brings the best out of you, develops well-formed maturity in you.

Mathew 6:33 MSG

If God gives such attention to the appearance of wildflowers—most of which are never seen—don't you think he'll attend to you, take pride in you, do his best for you? What I'm trying to do here is to get you to relax, to not be so preoccupied with getting, so you can respond to God's giving. People who don't know God and the way he works fuss over these things, but you know both God and how he works. Steep your life in God-reality, God-initiative, God-provisions. Don't worry about missing out. You'll find all your everyday human concerns will be met.

The two Bible passages above epitomize what a God-centered paradigm is all about. As you read in the previous chapters, your brain was processing large volumes of information. Your brain chooses what is important and what it discards. You actually retain or store only a small portion of the sensory information your brain receives. You remember the information and facts that you consider important. You are doing some of this consciously and much of it subconsciously.

You would be amazed if you knew the things that you miss or never perceive on a daily basis. I hope that the first chapter on paradigms convinced you on what you can miss as you live your life. You can change the way or manner in which you process the information your brain is receiving. You can change your paradigm through training on how you process the information. You think differently now than when you were younger. Adult brains still have tremendous plasticity. You can teach an old dog new tricks! You can start training your brain to perceive things in a different way. Just like people in the FBI who are trained to watch, listen, and perceive everything in their job or environment, Christians need to train themselves to perceive and understand what God is doing in this world. What is God doing in your life?

There were many times that God intervened in my life, but I did not pay attention to it or comprehend it. He was making sure that I would accomplish His plan that He has for me. The Bible says that He has a plan for every one of us. Developing a God-centered paradigm makes it easier to know and follow His plan for you.

In the Bible, many times the people of Israel failed to recognize or understand God's decrees or plans for them. There are many Bible verses that relate to that. Their hearts were hardened. They had ears, but they did not hear. They had eyes, but they did not see. That was their paradigm. God and Jesus were present right in front of them, but they failed to see them.

The question is how much are you missing? Has God been sending you signals, but you don't know it? Is Jesus knocking on the door waiting for you to hear Him?

2 Corinthians 4:4 NLT

Satan, who is the god of this world, has blinded the minds of those who don't believe. They are unable to see the glorious light of the Good News. They don't understand this message about the glory of Christ, who is the exact likeness of God.

You need to be very careful about what you believe you see or perceive. Satan is the great imitator or master of disguise. Sometimes you don't simply see something, because your paradigm keeps you from seeing. There are some things that are outside of your ability to see, such as things in the spiritual realm. Except in very unusual circumstances, man cannot see into the spiritual realm. But, you can improve your ability to see or perceive God in this world. It just takes practice and commitment.

There is a story or parable about a man who was trapped in his house during a flood. He began praying to God to rescue him. He had a vision in his head of God's hand reaching down from heaven and lifting him to safety. The water started to rise in his house. His neighbor urged him to leave and offered him a ride to safety. The man yelled back, "I am waiting for God to save me." So, the neighbor drove off in his pick-up truck.

The man continued to pray and hold on to his vision. As the water began rising in his house, he had to climb up to the roof. A boat came by with some people heading for safe ground. They yelled at the man to grab the rope they were ready to throw and take him to safety. He told them that he was waiting on God to save him. They shook their heads and moved on.

The man continued to pray, believing with all his heart that he would be saved by God. The flood waters continued to rise. A helicopter flew by. A voice came over a loud speaker offering to lower a ladder and take him off the roof. The man waved the helicopter away, shouting back that he was waiting for God to save him. The helicopter left.

The flooding water came over the roof and caught him up and swept him away. He drowned. When he reached heaven, he asked, "God, why did You not save me? I believed in You with all my heart. Why did you let me drown?"

God replied, "I sent you a pick-up truck, a boat, and a helicopter and you refused all of them. What else could I possibly do for you?"

Life is all about choices. The TV show *Let's Make a Deal* began in 1963. The show concludes with two contestants choosing between three doors. The suspense of the game is that you don't know what is behind the doors. It could be something as a fabulous vacation or a car. It could be what the show calls a Zonk, a worthless prize. Well, God is giving you the chance to pick one of three doors. The difference is that I am going to tell you what is behind each door.

Door 1

- Eternal life
- Up to 10 years or more of a longer, fuller, and healthier life on earth.
- A life filled with joy, peace, and love given by Jesus.
- A life full of the fruits of the Holy Spirit: love, joy, peace, patience, kindness, goodness, faithfulness, gentleness, and self-control.

Door 2
- A life of sitting on the fence or not excited about anything in life.
- A life like the people in Laodicea, whom God called lukewarm, stale, and stagnant.
- A life of just going through the motions.

Door 3 (Zonk)
- A life of sin which is destined to eternal damnation.
- A life based on who has the most toys at the end wins (but really loses).
- A life of partying, into self, all about me, me, me.
- A life of fear, worry, anger, anxiety, and depression.

Which door would you choose? Or you might think that you don't need to choose a door, but leave everything to chance. Leaving everything to chance leads to Door 3. Doing nothing and not purposely choosing a door or path in life is a choice. It's a very poor choice and leads to a life behind Door 3.

God wants everyone to choose Door 1. Once you have chosen Door 1, what's next? You need to center your life on the teachings of God. When you choose Door 1, you become a new creature. Just like the caterpillar, you turn into a beautiful butterfly. This is a paradigm shift or the paradigm shift of a lifetime.

What is the best way to fully and completely experience a new paradigm centered on God? As strange as it may seem, you need to start with a zero paradigm. The caterpillar becomes an amorphous mass of nothing and emerges as a beautiful butterfly. You are wondering, how do I do that? Experts in teaching paradigms and paradigm shifts know that this is the first step in the process of making changes. You have to start from scratch or zero.

I hope that from the first chapter on paradigms you now understand how paradigms work. You know that everything you perceive, understand, and the manner in which you react to everything in your life is directly related to your particular paradigm. Your paradigm is constantly changing. These changes are usually very slow, but a dramatic incident in your life can cause a large paradigm shift. Becoming a Christian is a huge paradigm shift. Now is the time to center your paradigm on God. A zero paradigm means you start from nothing. The life you lived before becoming a Christian is gone and over.

Isaiah 43:18 NIV

Forget the former things, do not dwell on the past.

You create a new paradigm by starting from zero. You make a list of characteristics that would be ideal or perfect for your new paradigm. The way you lived your life before has nothing to do with your new paradigm. Since we are thinking about a new God-centered paradigm, let's look at starting your paradigm as if God suddenly planted you on this earth. He tells you who He is, His son Jesus Christ had to be sacrificed as a pardon for your sins, and He has a plan for you to live your life by. You have no knowledge of your life before. What would you decide to do with your life? You start by making a list of characteristics of a person living a God-centered paradigm or life. Here is a list to think about. I am sure that you can think of others that you would like to add to your paradigm.

- Believe that God created the universe and you.
- God sent Jesus Christ to die for your sins.
- Believe that Jesus is your Lord and Savior.
- Welcome the Holy Spirit into your life.
- Study the Bible.
- Set up a daily prayer time.

- Attend church.
- Attend a Bible study.
- Be a member of a small group from your church.
- Volunteer at church.
- Have Christian friends.
- Enjoy Christian movies, books, TV, and radio. Every morning I listen to Christian radio on the way to work. It's a great way to start the day.
- Go on mission trips.
- Have a positive attitude.
- Receive and acknowledge the joy, peace, and love of Jesus Christ.
- Work on developing the fruits of the Holy Spirit.
- Begin a meditation program like the one in Chapter 14, which you do daily.
- Your soul and spirit need to be exercised, just like your body, in order to function at a high level.
- Attend a three-day Christian retreat such as: Great Banquet, Faith Walk, Cursillo, Cum Christo, Diaspora, Journey to Damascus, Tres Dias, Unidos en Cristo, Via de Cristo, Walk to Emmaus — Youth Retreats: Awakening, Chryalis, Happening — A Christian Experience, Vida Nueva, Vocare. (My experience at the Great Banquet was a fantastic way to get closer to God.)

You need to prioritize these and begin taking the time to incorporate them into your life. You have to make a God-centered paradigm a priority in your life. A God-centered paradigm will improve your health, as you read in the chapter on health. If you turn your life over to God, you will notice that stress, anxiety, worry, fear and doubt will begin to diminish. The meditation will start to calm your mind. God tells you not to worry and to believe that He is in charge of all things.

Now start down the path that God has planned for you. These are some steps for you to follow.

Perception

Learn to observe and perceive everything around you in your life. Perception is the key to understanding what God has in store for you. Train yourself to be more observant in all the things that happen in your life. You can do it just like FBI agents are trained to observe. Don't just look at things on the surface, but look deeper or from a different point of view.

Take a couple minutes twice a day just to observe what a fantastic and intricate world that God has made. Try to look at it differently. Observe things and circumstances in your life and how God may be working in those things. Maybe you watch a spider build a web or a bird building their nest. My favorite thing to do along this line is to go scuba diving. Like I mentioned earlier, I try to find a cleaning station—a car wash for grouper. Then I realize again, how truly amazing and how intricately God has designed and planned His world. Remember the videos I told you about in the chapter on paradigms, if you didn't watch them, watch them now.

God reveals himself in many different ways, if you take the time to look. I will cover a variety of other ways that God reveals himself to us that I believe you can contemplate as you go.

Jesus Christ

God revealed the magnitude of His love for you, when He was willing to sacrifice His son on the cross. Just thinking about that should make it easy for you to want to have your life centered on Him. Jesus brought light to a world of darkness. Search and seek that light and let His light shine through you.

Holy Spirit

The Holy Spirit gets left out sometimes when people discuss God. The Holy Spirit is your connection to God. God reveals Himself to you through His Spirit. The Holy Spirit is the key in developing a God-centered paradigm in your life. The relationship between your spirit and the Holy Spirit needs to be nurtured. That is where prayer and meditation can help. Make the Holy Spirit your best friend!

Prayer Life

You need to have an active prayer life. This is your chance to talk with God. God loves listening to your prayers. He is communicating with you all the time. Many times in this stress filled world, we don't hear Him or pay attention to Him. Spend time with God each day.

Christian Friends

Christian friends are very important to a God-centered paradigm. Remember that everything you see, hear, or observe can influence your paradigm. Spending time around people who don't share your same views can have an influence on you. Even if you don't believe what they say or do, it still can influence on you in a negative way. For the same reason, it is good to be around friends who have a positive attitude. As a Christian you are supposed to have a positive attitude.

Bible

The Bible reveals God's love to you. The Bible is the story of God's love for you. The Bible tells of His love and gives you instructions on how to live your life. It is a personal letter to you. Everything about life and what you need to know can be found in the Bible. Become a Bible expert. Read it daily.

Meditation

Read the Lord's charge to Joshua in Joshua 1:8-9. Study this Book of Instruction continually. Meditate on it day and night, so you will be sure to obey everything written in it. This is my command—be strong and courageous! Do not be afraid or discouraged. For the Lord your God is with you wherever you go.

Set up a time for meditation and devotion every day for thirty minutes. Follow the instructions in the previous chapter. As I listed before, there are so many benefits!

Galatians 5:22-23 NLT

But the Holy Spirit produces this kind of fruit in our lives: love, joy, peace, patience, kindness, goodness, faithfulness, gentleness, and self-control.

Through the Holy Spirit, work on developing the fruits of God's Spirit. Take each one at a time and work on how you can incorporate it into your life.

Joy

Joy is much different than being happy. Happy is a feeling that comes and goes. Joy is a state of mind which is unaffected by circumstances. Your soul is committed to God. It is the knowledge that God has you in His arms and you are under His care. You are in harmony with God.

Peace

So many people need to work through obtaining peace in their lives. It changes a person from a life of worry, fear, anxiety, and stress which leads to so much of the mental disease today. Peace comes with surrendering and yielding to God and giving Him control of your life. He is the creator of all things and He can obviously take care of you. Learn to relax, get in the passenger side of the car and let the Holy Spirit drive the car.

Patience

We need to practice the patience of Job. Patience means having endurance and perseverance through difficult times. There will always be difficult times in everyone's life. Remember, God is in control. Wait on Him.

Kindness

Kindness is being loving, caring, and benevolent to others. Christians should be the kindest people on earth. Can someone who sees you and your actions know that you are kind person? Can they tell you are a Christian without you having to tell them? Be kind.

Goodness

People who are good, do the right thing. They have integrity and are honest. They go the extra mile to help others.

Faithfulness

Being faithful is the glue that holds all this together. Faithful people are dependable and trustworthy. They value commitment as an important virtue. Do people trust you?

Gentleness

Your character is calming and soothing. You have a tender heart. People are comfortable in your presence.

Self-Control

Self-control is being obedient to God's laws and commands. You have discipline and restraint. When the tough get going, you are steady.

When the seas are rough, you are the captain at the control of your ship.

Love

I always leave this for last, when I talk about the fruits of the Spirit. For me, this is the most important fruit of all. God is love and God's love for us is beyond our limited ability to know how much. We are just simple beings that He created. Even though man has sinned over and over, turned away from Him, and done all kinds of things against Him, He still sent His one and only Son to save us. He loves us so much that His Son had to be treated in a brutally horrible manner and then take all the world's sins past, present, and future on Himself. We need to strive every day to emulate His love. How different the world would look if man learned to love!

Wake up every day and promise to be loving each day!

There are many more personal characteristics that a God-centered paradigm should have. There is a great list of these by Dr. Richard J. Krejcir which you can find at http://www.discipleshiptools.org.

Here some of the characteristics that I think should be a part of your God-centered paradigm:

Compassion, cooperativeness, thoughtfulness, diligent, honest, truthful, God is a priority, meekness, forgiving, fair, respectful, supportive, understanding, humility, agreeable, good example, role model, mentor, God's disciple, commitment, selfless, courage, reverent, dependable, perseverance, successful, friendship, gratitude, attentiveness, conviction, holiness, discretion, devotion, and just.

How many of these characteristics would your friends or family use to describe you? Take time to think about how you can improve on each of the characteristics above. If there are some that you may not feel are a description of you, make a list and begin to incorporate them into your life.

Here is a list of actions you that can start:

1. Make God a priority.
2. God is a God of love.
3. Read the Bible daily.
4. Pray daily.
5. Meditation daily (You can do 3, 4, and 5 at same time—30 minutes)
6. Moderate exercise at least 4 days a week (brisk walk is OK—30 minutes)

7. Mediterranean diet, green salad for one meal a day, limit animal protein to 4 ounces a day.
8. Active in all aspects of church.
9. No stress, no anxiety, don't worry, no fear, and forgive yourself and others. (Turn everything over to God.)
10. Give to others and volunteer.
11. Good night's sleep.
12. Practice looking at things and circumstances from a different point of view. (Train yourself on your perception techniques.)
13. Set short term and long term goals.

You need to follow Jesus' new commandment. Love the Lord God with all your heart, all your soul, all your strength, and all your mind. God loves you beyond His commandment to you. Love your neighbor as you love yourself.

Deuteronomy 4:9 NLT

But watch out! Be careful never to forget what you yourself have seen. Do not let those memories escape from your mind as long as you live! And be sure to pass them on to your children and grandchildren.

God is telling you throughout the Bible that He wants you to learn to become more sensitive to the presence of His Spirit that cannot be seen or perceived under everyday simple methods. Through His Spirit, you become a new creature. Your soul, spirit, heart, and mind are changed. After Moses was in the presence of God, he looked different. Moses' face shined from the presence of God.

Jesus Christ is the light unto the world. You will shine as well, as you are Jesus' disciple. Even though you may feel that your light is small and dim, light will always fill darkness. If you remember, I told you that the eye could see a single candle in darkness 30 miles away. Darkness is the absence of anything or energy. There is much darkness in this world today. Every shining light no matter how small can bring light to someone. Light always wins over darkness.

Being a shining light reminds me of a story about the hymn, *Thy Word*. The hymn is based on Psalm 119:105 NLT.

Your word is a lamp unto my feet and a light for my path.

Thy Word is song written by Amy Grant and her co-worker Michael W. Smith. Michael says that he came up with the melody and some of the words from the book of Psalms. Michael wasn't sure about the words of the song and gave it to Amy to finish. She struggled with it for a few days. She was in Maine where the nights were cold and very dark. Amy left the studio to go back to her cabin. She became completely lost. There are bears, moose, and mountain lions in the forest there. Out in the distance she saw a small light. She stumbled and followed her way to the light. It was a lantern in her cabin window. She went inside and sat down. She couldn't believe what had just happened. She wrote the words to the song which included *Thy word is a lamp unto my feet, and a light unto my path.*

Shift your paradigm to one that is centered on God. Meditate and live thinking about the joy, peace, happiness, and love that has been given to you by Jesus Christ. Become a shining light.

I hope that reading this book has revealed to you that your brain and eyes are designed in a fabulous way. Even still, you miss many of the things happening in your life. Your brain is making new brains cells constantly. It is not just sitting there passing time. Train yourself to perceive things in a new way. Make changing your paradigm a fun thing. Learning new things should be interesting and fun.

As in the parable of the prodigal son, the father saw his son coming home far out in the distance. He did not wait for his son to come to the house. He ran to his son, embraced him, kissed him, and held a great feast in his honor. God is running to you. Can you see Him? Are you running to Him? Don't miss Him!

A God-Centered Paradigm (Life) Place Your Life Before God

Get your new paradigm. God is waiting!

**May God bless you on your journey
through this life on your way home to Him.**

Epilogue

I hope that you have enjoyed reading this book and have found it to be a blessing. Paradigms are an interesting subject. Everything that you see, perceive, hear, or think you understand is based on your paradigm and/or experiences. People's paradigms can be very rigid and narrow. They miss many things in their lives, as if they have tunnel vision. Or like some horses running in a race, they have blinders on so they can't see any of the other horses.

This book was an attempt to show you how expanding or thinking outside the box can lead to a new life. God is present everywhere. Most of us don't take the time to observe Him in our everyday lives. The Bible is full of instances where God's people failed to perceive or understand God's plan for them. That failed perception is still going on today. The Bible is the ultimate source for developing your paradigm.

The Bible is a love story about God's love for you. The Bible gives you instructions and laws about living life. The *United States Constitution* is based on the laws in the Bible, though it seems like the Supreme Court over the last several years is trying to change the current laws. The Bible gives you advice and instruction on your diet, sanitation, health, mental health, and all the aspects for living your life.

The secular world and Satan, as it says in Romans 12:2, want you to *conform* to their ways. You have to be politically correct. It is all about me. Money and power are what is important. God is not supposed to be out in the public arena, no prayer in schools, keep your religion to yourself, and on and on. Society is on a downward spiral in America and

God is getting pushed out of our nation. We can't have the word *God* in our Pledge of Allegiance. God cannot be in our schools. People have taken President Jefferson's private letter about separation of church and state out of context. It was never in the Constitution. But, God says we are not to conform to the ways of the world, but to transform and continually renew our minds on things that God wants us to do.

In the health care field, God has a plan for you. Nearly all the diets that have been written are people's opinions. Many times they don't have good medical evidence to support them. The Mediterranean diet has been thoroughly studied and it compares to the recommendation by God in the Bible. We were originally designed to be vegetarians. You should try to limit the amount of animal protein that you eat per day. You don't have to be a fitness fanatic to be healthy, but moderate exercise four days a week is important. Light weight training or the use of bands is beneficial for good muscle tone. The blue zones around the world did not just happen, there are diet and lifestyle reasons for those people living longer and being healthier. There are many sources for diet plans based on the Mediterranean diet. You should eat a green salad with nuts, fruits, and seeds for one meal each day and be careful about what dressing you are putting on the salad. The dressing can change a healthy salad to a horrible meal full of bad calories.

Stress, anxiety, fear, worry, anger, and other negative emotions are the leading cause of physical and mental health issues people face today. There is a basis for stress as a cause or contributing factor for nearly all the diseases that are killing people today. All these negative emotions release large amounts of free radicals into your body, which is not healthy. Truly turning your life over to God, results in letting God help you with those emotions.

With everyone being bombarded with the garbage on TV, social media, music, Hollywood, and other forms of media, it is no wonder that people are having trouble controlling their limbic systems and emotions. This is especially true for children. You should monitor what they are watching, the video games they are playing, and their activity on social media.

If you get an impulse from your limbic system to do something you know is wrong or sinful, eat a food that is not healthy, get emotionally upset about something, or other negative thought, think *what would I do if Jesus were standing here?* Maybe pick a favorite Bible verse such as Philippians 4:13. For *I can do all things through Christ, who gives me strength.* You can try taking a few slow deep breaths if you are upset. If you are having significant emotional problems, seek the help of your pastor or Christian counselor, psychologist, or psychiatrist.

Technology now allows us to see how God effects brain function. God changes the way your brain functions. Christians have been shown to have larger brains. We now know that your brain is constantly forming new brain cells, even when you are older. You do have the ability to change your life. Just like the caterpillar that turns into a beautiful butterfly, you can have, not a partial metamorphosis, but a complete metamorphosis.

When you become a Christian, you become a new creature. You start making millions of new brains cells connected to God. The more time you spend studying, praying, and meditating on the Bible and God, the brain becomes stronger, as you are making God-centered neurons. The old sinful neurons will be gradually removed or pruned from your brain by not using those circuits.

God breathed into man His spirit and soul. It is still a mystery about how the brain thinks, its conscience, and how your decision making processes work. Once you become a Christian, the Holy Spirit resides in your brain. The key to life is letting the Holy Spirit be your tour guide. God is all about love, as you see in the life of Jesus. God wants you to live a long, healthy, joyful, peaceful, and loving life. God wants you to be successful, help others, grow the fruits of the Spirit, and follow His plan that He has for you. The best way to accomplish it is to have a God-centered paradigm.

Epilogue

I recently heard a sermon by Brad Rogers, who is one of our pastors. The title of his sermon was *Facetime*. God wants Facetime with you. There are many instances in the Bible which talks about face to face time with God. You can find some of these in Exodus 33:11 with Moses, Genesis 32:30 concerning Jacob, Judges 6:22 with Gideon, Psalm 27:8 with King David, and Paul talks about it in 1 Corinthians 13:12. The question is, Do you or are you able to have Facetime with God? Does your paradigm allow you to perceive or understand God communicating with you? My prayer is that this book has helped you with making God the center of your paradigm and has brought you closer to Him. You are able to see Him working in your life and you communicate with Him daily.

If this book has helped you become a new follower of Christ, there are some resources that will help you begin your journey. You can Google *The Four Spiritual Laws*. There are the DVDs *The Wonders of God's Creation*. You can search on YouTube for *God of Wonders-The Documentary*. You should find a good Bible-based church and seek assistance there, as well.

Make God a priority and start the steps listed in Chapter 15. Give the plan three months and see if your life isn't different. I am sure that God wants you to be closer to Him. I pray that this book and its approach to living a God-centered paradigm will be a blessing to you. You might be surprised by what you find you are missing or not perceiving in your life.

God has a big smile on His face, His arms are wide open, and He can't wait to be involved in everything you do.

Just trust, see, perceive, and let go to start your journey to a God-centered paradigm.

God Bless You!

About the Author

Dr. Croley made the decision to become an ophthalmologist at age 14. He felt a calling to help people with their vision. He has spent his life working and researching in the field of eye care. Dr. Croley has been practicing ophthalmology for over 35 years in Southwest Florida.

Dr. Croley has served on numerous boards and committees of the American Academy of Ophthalmology, Florida Society of Ophthalmology, Bonita Springs Lions Eye Clinic, and others. He has served as President of the Florida Society of Ophthalmology. Dr. Croley developed a telemedicine computer system in the 1990s when very few people knew about telemedicine. He also developed an electronic medical records program that he has used in his office since 1998. Seeing the need for funding for the local center that takes care of the blind called The Lighthouse for the Blind, he began its original fundraiser for the organization.

In addition to his passion for helping people see better, Dr. Croley uses his love of gourmet cooking to support local charities by inviting people into his home and preparing gourmet dinners with all the proceeds benefiting charities.

He lectures on eye diseases, teaches courses on eye surgery and eye disease treatments. He lectures at churches and various groups about subjects related to this book.

CPSIA information can be obtained
at www.ICGtesting.com
Printed in the USA
FSOW04n0256081216
28259FS